Genetics and Psychopharmacology

Modern Problems of Pharmacopsychiatry

Vol. 10

Series Editors:
Th.A. Ban, Montreal, Que.
F.A. Freyhan, Washington, D.C.
P. Pichot, Paris
W. Pöldinger, Wil/St. Gallen

S. Karger · Basel · München · Paris · London · New York · Sydney

Genetics and Psychopharmacology

Volume Editor:
J. Mendlewicz, Brussels/New York, N.Y.

With 15 figures and 25 tables, 1975

S. Karger · Basel · München · Paris · London · New York · Sydney

Modern Problems of Pharmacopsychiatry

Vol. 1–4: Details on request
Vol. 5: The Neuroleptics
    X + 190 p., 38 fig., 9 tab., 1970. ISBN 3–8055–0530–2
Vol. 6: The Role of Drugs in Community Psychiatry
    VI + 128 p., 3 fig., 3 tab., 1971. ISBN 3–8055–1200–7
Vol. 7: Psychological Measurements in Psychopharmacology
    VI + 267 p., 25 fig., 54 tab., 1974. ISBN 3–8055–1630–4
Vol. 8: Psychotropic Drugs and the Human EEG
    X + 377 p., 95 fig., 19 tab., 1974. ISBN 3–8055–1419–0
Vol. 9: Trazodone
    VI + 210 p., 86 fig., 83 tab., 1974. ISBN 3–8055–1781–1

Cataloging in Publication
Genetics and psychopharmacology
Volume editor: J. Mendlewicz. Basel, New York, Karger, 1975
(Modern problems of pharmacopsychiatry, v. 10)
1. Pharmacogenetics 2. Psychopharmacology
I. Mendlewicz, J., ed. II. Title III Series
W1 MO168P v.10/QV 77 R295
ISBN 3–8055–2117–0

© Copyright 1975 by S. Karger AG, Basel (Switzerland), Arnold-Böcklin-Strasse 25
Printed in Switzerland by Thür AG Offsetdruck, Pratteln
ISBN 3–8055–2117–0

Contents

Introduction

The rates of metabolism of drugs vary significantly between different individuals. However, within the same individual, this rate appears to be quite constant. Twin and family studies indicate that interindividual variations in rates of drug biotransformation are to a large extent determined by genetic rather than environmental factors. This phenomenon has been demonstrated for various drugs such as imipramine, nortriptyline, phenylbutazone, ethanol, diphenylhydantoin and others and is important in understanding differences in drug response. Pharmacogenetics is a relatively new field which originates from the study of clinical consequences of hereditary variation in the handling of drugs as exemplified by the glucose-6-phosphate dehydrogenase deficiency. This syndrome is determined by genes located on the X chromosome and is clinically expressed by hemolysis when a susceptible individual is exposed to several drugs. The field of pharmacogenetics is now being extended to the study of polymorphic systems in man (such as the pseudocholinesterase polymorphism and the INH-acetyltransferase polymorphism) and also to the therapy of genetic disorders. There are a number of genetically determined disorders that are caused by enzyme deficiencies for which etiology and treatment have been illuminated by classical genetic and biochemical studies. This has some important implications for understanding the pathogenesis of such diseases as schizophrenia, manic-depressive illness and epilepsy, in which genetic factors have been shown to play an important role. Enzymes such as dopamine β-hydroxylase and monoamine oxidase regulate the intracellular and extracellular metabolism of several biogenic amines which have been hypothesized to play a role in the pathogenesis of major psychiatric disorders. These enzymes are known to be genetically determined to a large extent and are the subject of psychiatric investigations as indicated by this monograph. Recent developments in psychopharmacology described in this volume also indicate that depressive patients show genetic differences in their response rate to psychoactive drugs such as lithium carbonate, the tricyclics, and the MAO inhibitors. Environmental factors are also shown to interact with the genetic mechanisms underlying drug metabolism and drug response and the study of this interaction is of crucial importance for understanding and treating psychiatric disorders.

J. Mendlewicz

Genetics and Psychopharmacology. Mod. Probl. Pharmacopsych., vol. 10, pp. 1–11, ed. *J. Mendlewicz*, Brussels (Karger, Basel 1975)

Relationship of Genetic Factors to Course and Drug Response in Schizophrenia, Mania and Depression[1]

George Winokur

Department of Psychiatry, University of Iowa College of Medicine, Iowa City, Iowa

The ability to alter the natural history of chronic or remitting illness must be present if the drug is to be considered effective. In the schizophrenias and affective disorders we know a considerable amount about the short- and long-term course of the illnesses. These kinds of data are obtained in systematic follow-up studies. A follow-up study is important for two reasons. It tells whether an illness goes on to chronicity or the illness remits and never recurs, or the illness remits and has recurrences over time. Illnesses may be categorized as to whether they are remitting or chronic. This is of considerable importance in the differentiation of schizophrenia from the affective disorders. The follow-up of illness may be evaluated in both a social and medical context. The social context would be concerned with whether or not the patient is functioning in a viable fashion in the community. A medical context would be concerned with whether or not the patient manifests the symptoms of a particular disease.

There is, however, another and perhaps even more important reason for a follow-up. Over the course of time a highly relevant question is whether an illness will change its characteristics and begin to fulfill the criteria for the diagnosis of another and different illness. Thus, it is important to know whether affective disorder patients in the long run could show the clinical characteristics of schizophrenia. If depressives and manics never show the end states of schizophrenia, it strengthens the evidence that the affective disorders should be considered as totally different kinds of illnesses than schizophrenia. Likewise, it is important to know whether the use of any therapeutic modality would alter the clinical picture in such a way as to make it appear as a different disease.

1   This work was supported in part by USPHS Grant No. MH24189.

Genetic factors have been studied to a large extent in both the schizophrenias and the affective disorders. It is possible to assess the relationship of these factors to the course of the illness. The roles of specific genetic backgrounds in their relationship to the results of pharmacotherapy, however, is a virtually untouched field.

To obtain agreement that schizophrenia and the affective disorders are distinct entities and different from each other, one should have clear evidence that there are correlations between symptom picture, follow-up, family history and response to treatment within each diagnostic group. A proper study would include data on all 4 of the variables in the *same* group of patients. Generally, however, most studies deal with only two variables and one has to adopt the euclidean axiom that things equal to the same thing are equal to each other in order to fulfill the correlative possibilities. There is considerable material on clinical picture, family history and course. Data on the fourth variable, response to treatment, are skimpy, particularly as regards the relationships with family history; but there are a few studies which are relevant to schizophrenia and the affective disorders. The purpose of this paper is to discuss these variables and present data on their relationships.

Clinical Picture, Course, Family History in Schizophrenics versus Manics versus Depressives

A recent study encompasses a systematic evaluation of patients, a blind follow-up from records and a blind family history from records. 525 patients were chosen according to strict criteria and were placed into one of 3 groups (1–3). Thus, 200 schizophrenics, 100 manics and 225 depressives entered as part of a large study. The records on these patients were extremely complete and contained extensive follow-up and family history data. Table I presents differences in the clinical picture at the time of index admission. Though the criteria which were used to select patients would influence the evaluation of the clinical picture, no single symptom would separate or exclude any particular patient from entering one of these 3 groups. It is clear from table I that clinical pictures are quite different.

The blind family history is presented in table II. Few differences were seen between manics and depressives; something which should not be surprising as the patients were generally rated as having relatives with a remitting disorder or chronic disorder. No effort was made to evaluate the relatives in terms of whether they had manias and/or depressions, *per se*. Of considerable importance is the fact that in the first-degree family groups (of affective disorders versus schizophrenics) there are clear differences for both familial schizophrenia and affective disorder. The differential for the extended family (maternal and pater-

Table I. Clinical characteristics of schizophrenics, manics and depressives

	Schizo-phrenics	Manics	Depres-sives
Number studied	200	100	225
Age of onset (median), years	26	27	39
Weight loss, %	7	12	39
Energy loss, %	23	11	70
Terminal insomnia, %	2	12	18
Euphoric or irritable, %	2	94	0
Extravagance, %	2	19	0
Social withdrawal, %	72	3	32
Primary delusions, %	25	4	4
Persecutory delusions, %	42	25	17
Auditory hallucinations, %	54	15	6
Haptic hallucinations, %	29	5	8
Motor symptoms (tics, stereotypies, verbigerations, grimacing, waxy flexibility, posturing), %	32	11	2

Table II. Familial (genetic) background in schizophrenics versus affective disorder patients

Morbid risks for parents and sibs

Probands	affective disorder, %	schizophrenia, %
Schizophrenics (N = 200)	5.5 ⎤ p < 0.0005	2.1 ⎤ p < 0.005
Affective disorders (N = 325) (100 manics, 235 depressives)	13.5 ⎦	0.6 ⎦

Proportion with extended family history of:

	affective disorder, %	schizophrenia, %	alcoholism, %
Schizophrenics	17.5	6.5	15
Affective disorder	18.4	3.1	5.9

Suicides in parents and sibs of probands with:

affective disorder, %	schizophrenia, %
3	1

nal sides) is less reliable and the affective disorder finding in both groups is almost equal. Any single family could be counted only once even if it had many members with affective disorder in it; and because of the high prevalence of affective disorder in the general population an extended family history of affective disorder is not particularly useful in differentiating the affective disorders from schizophrenia. On the other hand, the extended families of schizophrenics were over twice as likely to show schizophrenia than the extended families of the affective disorders. The differences between extended families on the variable of alcoholism is highly significant ($p < 0.0005$) but uninterpretable at present.

The usefulness of the family history may now be seen in the follow-up material which is presented in table III. It is important to know that both the follow-up and the family history were done independently and blindly as to the diagnosis or each other. The patient with affective disorder in a family history and who was diagnosed as having affective disorder himself is likely to have a remitting illness. A schizophrenic patient is likely to have a family history of schizophrenia and to have himself a chronic unremitting disorder which tends towards deterioration. Thus, the family history of schizophrenia would in fact predict a downhill course and a family history of affective disorder could be used to predict a remission.

These patients were admitted to a hospital between 1934 and 1944, long before the advent of effective drug therapy or even electroshock therapy. As a consequence, no material is available on response to treatment. However, it is of considerable importance that there is a clustering of specific factors: follow-up, family history and clinical picture. Any one of these factors could reliably predict any of the others.

In a general sense, familial findings would predict response to treatment. There is no reason to believe that antidepressant medication is of any significant value in changing the course of nuclear schizophrenia and, thus, a family history of nuclear schizophrenia would predict poor response to this kind of treatment. On the other hand, the use of phenothiazines which are of value in chronic

Table III. Course (follow-up) in schizophrenics manics, and depressives

	Schizo-phrenics %	Manics %	Depres-sives %
Discharged to community	26	39	48
Ever recovered in follow-up	8	54	59
Never remitted in follow-up	78	21	20
Deteriorated	13	0	2
Continuously hospitalized after 10 years follow-up	19	0	0

schizophrenia might also be of value in mania; and as a consequence neither the presence nor the absence of a family history of schizophrenia or affective disorder should predict very much about the value of phenothiazines in the affective disorders (manias and depressions) taken as a broad group. However, as will be apparent from the following section, the affective disorders are divisible into major types and a family history of a particular sort might well be relevant to predicting the usefulness of specific drug therapy in affective disorder.

Bipolar versus Unipolar Affective Disorder, Genetic Factors Course and Drug Response

In 1966, the affective disorders were separated on the basis of a specific family history into two major groups, bipolar affective disorder (manias only or manias and depression) and unipolar illness (depression only). Starting with groups of patients who have shown a mania and comparing them to patients who have shown only depressions, extremely striking differences are found, both in the family history and in the course of illness (4—6). Table IV presents some of the differences.

Likewise, there now appear to be specific drug effects which are related to these particular findings. Lithium in the acute treatment of a depression appears to be more effective if the person has bipolar illness than if the person has simple depressive disease (7, 8). Thus, a family history of mania in a patient would suggest more success in the acute treatment of depression than if such a family history finding were absent.

A report of a large US Veterans Administration-National Institute of Mental Health (VA-NIMH) collaborative study group project on the use of lithium carbonate and imipramine in the prevention of affective episodes has recently been evaluated and published (9). Bipolar patients were particularly striking because of the fact that lithium was significantly more effective than either

Table IV. Differences in familial pathology and course in manics versus depressives

	Manics	Depressives
Age of onset, years	28	36
Biphasic or triphasic immediate course	yes	no
Relapse in 2 years after index admission, %	61	48
Episodes prior to index admission per person	3.5	0.9
Well in every way in 6-year follow-up, %	7	34
Affective disorder in at least one parent, %	52	26
Morbid risk for mania in first-degree family members, %	14	0.29—0.35

imipramine or placebo in preventing subsequent affective attacks of such severity that they would require hospitalization or other kinds of treatment. This study fulfills almost all of the requirements that were mentioned above in the introduction. The family history, the clinical picture, the course on placebo and the course on effective drug were all studied at the same time and in the same group of patients. A family history of mania would predict a clinical picture of bipolar illness which, in turn, would predict increased efficacy of preventing affective episodes over the long run.

In the VA-NIMH study there was a suggestion that imipramine might precipitate manic episodes in bipolar patients. In unipolar patients prevention of affective episodes was related to treatment with either lithium or imipramine; both treatments were more effective than placebo. Of importance is the fact that in this study the family history of the unipolar and bipolar patients was quite different. Bipolar affective illness was found in 9 % of the relatives of the bipolar group and 0 % of the relatives of the unipolar group. Unipolar relatives have only 19 % unipolar affective illness; bipolar relatives had 36 % of unipolar affective illness. Thus, there is a relationship of the family history findings to both course and treatment in the 2 groups.

It is possible that bipolar illness is, in itself, a heterogeneous entity; if this were true, a specific family history could be related to both differences in course and effect of treatment. *Mendlewicz et al.* examined a large number of manic-depressive patients and followed them over time (10). They conducted a blind study of bipolar patients on lithium and placebo. To enter the study, the patients had to have been normothymic and to have been followed for at least 6 months. Taking only their lithium group (N = 36) they found that responders to lithium in the follow-up period were significantly more likely ($p < 0.05$) to have a positive first-degree family history of bipolar illness. If both first- and second-degree relatives are taken into account, there was even a more significant association ($p < 0.01$) of response to lithium therapy and a positive family history for bipolar illness. *Taylor and Abrams* (11) have also collected data which would be in favor of heterogeneity in manic-depressive disease. Early-onset (before 30 years) patients were differentiated from late-onset patients in that first-degree relatives of the former had more affective illness and associated conditions (alcoholism, drug abuse and sociopathy). The early-onset patients had a bipolar course (depressions and manias); the late-onset patients tended to have only manias. Thus, a family history of a specific sort may be associated with both response to treatment and other aspects of the course of the illness.

A potentially valuable methodology to determine the influence of genetic factors on response to treatment and course would be to examine the effect of various drugs in family members who manifest the same illness. This is not an area of any great depth, but *Angst* (12) collected 14 related pairs, both of whom who had been treated with imipramine. In 9 of the pairs the effectiveness of this drug was the same in both members but in 5 pairs the drug was effective in one member and ineffective in the other. One of the problems in this evaluation was that some of the pair members had schizophrenic diagnoses whereas others had diagnoses of affective disorder. If the case material was grouped according to patients suffering from depression only, 9 of the 14 pairs were available. In this case 8 of the 9 revealed a similar response. In 5 of the 9 pairs imipramine had a good effect; and in 3 it was a failure; and in one pair one member responded well and the other poorly. *Angst* himself points out that it would be difficult to assume that the similarity in drug response could be attributed to blood relationship. In fact, it might be that the psychopathological picture and course were similar and the response might have been due to other than drug-induced factors. One of the 14 pairs was composed of monozygotic twin sisters, one of whom was diagnosed as having depressive schizophrenia and the other as having paranoid schizophrenia. Both twins were paranoid. One twin had a successful response to imipramine, the other did not. However, in neither case did the paranoid symptoms remit. *Pare* (13) also studied response to medication in related persons. He compared ill probands to ill relatives on the responses to differing groups of antidepressants. Though his material is small he found that probands and their ill relatives tended to respond to the same drugs, a point which suggested to him that perhaps more than one biochemical abnormality might account for depressive illnesses and that each one was genetically specific.

Pharmacogenetic Factors in Affective Illness

It is entirely possible that a drug which is sometimes effective in the treatment of an illness will *only* be effective if the drug is metabolized in a particular way. The metabolism of many drugs may well be relevant to genetic factors which have no relationship at all to the illness for which the drug is used. In a large group of patients who have a specific psychiatric disorder, only those patients who have special kinds of drug metabolism will respond to a particular treatment. This may be of some importance in the treatment of the affective disorders.

Johnstone and Marsh (14) recently studied the effect of phenelzine, a monoamine oxidase inhibitor, in 72 patients with 'neurotic depression'. Fast or slow acetylation of a monoamine oxidase inhibitor is a genetic polymorphism. These investigators found that improvement over 6 weeks was significantly greater in those patients who were slow acetylators. Phenelzine was no more efficacious than placebo in fast acetylators.

However, *Price Evans et al.* (15) present data on 47 depressed patients which open these findings to question. The *Price Evans* study divided depressed patients into 'neurotic' and 'endogenous' types and into fast and slow acetylator phenotypes. There were no significant differences in improvement between the 2 phenotypes, but slow acetylators showed more severe adverse effects to the phenelzine than the fast acetylators.

Åsberg et al. (16) studied the relationship of plasma level of nortriptyline to therapeutic effects. Amelioration of depression was related to an intermediate plasma level. With the lower and higher plasma levels, amelioration was unusual. Confirmation of the lack of therapeutic effect of high plasma levels of nortriptyline has recently been published (17). The steady-state plasma level of nortriptyline is most probably under genetic control. Data which support this have been reported by *Alexanderson et al.* (18), who studied 19 monozygotic twins and 20 dizygotic twins between the ages of 45 and 51 years. In monozygotic twins who were not treated with other drugs, there was considerable intra-pair similarity in plasma concentrations of nortriptyline; this intrapair similarity was not found in fraternal twins. A pedigree study by *Åsberg et al.* (19) supports a genetic factor in nortriptyline metabolism and suggests polygenetic inheritance. Though the control of plasma levels of nortriptyline certainly seems to be under genetic control, the relationship of this plasma level to clinical efficacy is still open to question. Thus, *Burrows et al.* (20) found no significant positive relationship between clinical response and plasma levels in 2 studies. They suggest, however, that studies of some individual patients might show this kind of relationship; therefore, studies should be related to those patients who do, in fact, respond to antidepressant medication with amelioration.

A pharmacogenetic finding of great importance to the field of psychiatry and, in particular, to the affective disorders is related to pseudocholinesterase deficiency. Some homozygous persons have an atypical pseudocholinesterase which is low in activity (21). When given a muscle relaxant such as suxamethonium these persons suffer from a prolonged apnea and if breathing is not accomplished for them it is quite possible that they will die. As muscle relaxants are used often in electroshock treatment a certain number of patients are at risk for this prolonged apnea. Though such patients are few, they are subject to a potentially tragic outcome because of abnormal metabolism of the muscle relaxant.

Schizophrenia

Though the literature is rife with comments about the possibility that schizophrenia is composed of more than one entity, this remains unproven. Certainly there are marked differences in clinical pictures of patients called schizophrenic. This could be due to the possibility of heterogeneity within the diagnosis; it could also be the result of polygenic transmission. In a polygenic transmission a more severe form of the illness would contain more of the genes

Table V. Differences between paranoid and hebephrenic schizophrenics

Symptoms	Hebephrenic	Paranoid
Symbolism, %	20	41
Tangentiality, %	57	20
Motor symptoms, %	36	12
Inappropriate affect, %	19	6
Follow-up (2–10⁺ years)		
Complete recovery, %	9	30
Held a job after index admission, %	23	70
Family history		
Proportion of relatives schizophrenic, %	2.4	0.8

but there would be a common genetic background for both the more and less severe types. Table V indicates that there are marked differences between hebephrenic and paranoid schizophrenia. These data come from a systematic clinical follow-up and family study (22, 23). The differences in clinical picture as well as the differences in follow-up material are statistically significant. Though there is a 3-fold increase of schizophrenia in the hebephrenic families compared to the paranoid families this finding in table V is not significant. Nevertheless, *Kallman*'s material (24) on children of schizophrenic indicates that twice as many children of hebephrenic probands (17.3 %) are ill with schizophrenia as opposed to the children of paranoid probands (8.5 %). *Shultz*'s material (25) on siblings is likewise in favor of an increase in schizophrenia in siblings of hebephrenics compared to siblings of paranoids.

Deterioration, defined as a difficulty in communicating, an inability to care for one's self and inability to work were seen in 2 of 23 paranoids (9 %) in a follow-up period of 4.3 years but in 10 of 56 hebephrenics (18 %) followed for a period of 4.6 years. It seems clear that the hebephrenic type of illness has a worse prognosis than the paranoid type. In addition hebephrenics have more schizophrenia in the family than paranoids.

Hebephrenia is associated with more thought disorder and more affective change. Motor symptoms are seen more in hebephrenic schizophrenia than in paranoid schizophrenia; one must question whether or not the differentiation between hebephrenic and catatonic schizophrenia of a chronic type is really possible. Suffice it to say, that the impairment of the hebephrenic schizophrenic leads to more inertia, more avolition and more lack of initiative. These are the so-called 'negative' symptoms of the illness. Whether they are the result of chronic hospitalization or an end point of illness process is unknown at this point. Once seen, however, these negative symptoms are unlikely to respond to treatment with the phenothiazine drugs. A study by *Letemendia and Harris* (26) on the use of chlorpromazine in chronic schizophrenic patients indicated unresponsiveness to medication in those patients in whom the chronic defect states appeared prominently as a lack of initiative. It is, thus, entirely possible that 4 things clustered together — a chronic defect state associated with avolition and a diagnosis of hebephrenic or catatonic schizophrenia, an increase in family history of schizophrenia and an unresponsiveness to the usual medication which is given to patients with schizophrenia.

Conclusions

There are significant findings in the areas of clinical picture, course, family history and drug response in both schizophrenia and the various affective disorders. Few studies have been done of similarly ill family members who might respond to one drug used for a particular illness but not to another. Pharmacogenetics has turned out to be a possibly productive field in helping predict response to drugs in various psychiatric illnesses. For the clinician it would appear that a knowledge of family history and family background may well be of considerable importance in making a diagnosis and suggesting a course of treatment. If family members show the same kinds of illnesses as do the probands, the family members have at least had an opportunity to be observed for a period of time; and, thus, unlike the case of the probands the clinician knows the course of their illness. This can be of considerable value in making decisions about the patient himself.

References

1 *Morrison, J.; Clancy, J.; Crowe, R., and Winokur, G.:* The Iowa 500. Diagnostic validity in mania, depression, and schizophrenia. Arch. gen. Psychiat. *27:* 457–461 (1972).
2 *Winokur, G.; Morrison, J.; Clancy, J., and Crowe, R.:* The Iowa 500. A blind family history comparison in mania, depression and schizophrenia. Arch. gen. Psychiat. *27:* 462–464 (1972).
3 *Morrison, J.; Winokur, G.; Crowe, R., and Clancy, J.:* The Iowa 500. The first follow-up. Arch. gen. Psychiat. *29:* 678–682 (1973).
4 *Winokur, G.; Clayton, P., and Reich, T.:* Manic depression illness (Mosby, St. Louis 1969).
5 *Angst, J. and Perris, C.:* Nosology of endogenous depression, a comparison of the findings of two studies. Z. ges. Neurol. Psychiat. *210:* 273 (1968).
6 *Perris, C.* (ed.): A study of bipolar (manic-depressive) and unipolar recurrent depressive psychoses. Acta psychiat. scand. *42:* suppl. 194, p. 1 (1966).
7 *Noyes, R.; Dempsey, G.; Blum, A., and Cavanaugh, G.:* Lithium treatment of depression. Comp. Psychiat. (in press).
8 *Goodwin, F.; Murphy, D.; Dunner, D., and Bunney, W.:* Lithium response in unipolar versus bipolar depression. Amer. J. Psychiat. *129:* 44–47 (1972).

9 *Prien, R.; Klett, J., and Caffey, E.:* Lithium carbonate and imipramine in prevention of affective episodes. Arch. gen. Psychiat. *29:* 420–425 (1973).
10 *Mendlewicz, J.; Fieve, R., and Stallone, F.:* Relationship between the effectiveness of lithium therapy and family history. Amer. J. Psychiat. *130:* 1011–1013 (1973).
11 *Taylor, M. and Abrams, R.:* Manic states. A genetic study of early and late onset affective disorders. Arch. gen. Psychiat. *28: 656* 660 (1973).
12 *Angst, J.:* A clinical analysis of the effects of tofranil in depression. Psychopharmacology *2:* 381–407 (1961).
13 *Pare, C.:* Differentiation of two genetically specific types of depression by the response to antidepressant drugs. Humangenetik *9:* 199–201 (1970).
14 *Johnstone, E. and Marsh, W.:* Acetylator status and response to phenelzine in depressed patients. Lancet *i:* 567–570 (1973).
15 *Price Evans, D.; Davison, K., and Pratt, R.:* The influence of acetylator phenotype on the effects of treating depression with phenelzine. Clin. Pharmacol. Ther. *6:* 430–435 (1965).
16 *Åsberg, M.; Crönholm, B.; Sjöqvist, F., and Tuck, D.:* Relationship between plasma level and therapeutic effect of nortriptyline. Brit. med. J. *iii:* 331–334 (1971).
17 *Kragh-Sørensen, L.P.; Hansen, C., and Åsberg, M.:* Plasma levels of nortriptyline in the treatment of endogenous depression. Acta psychiat. scand. *49:* 444–456 (1973).
18 *Alexanderson, B.; Price Evans, D., and Sjöqvist, F.:* Steady state plasma levels of nortriptyline in twins. Influence of genetic factors and drug therapy. Brit. med. J. *iv:* 764–768 (1969).
19 *Åsberg, M.; Price Evans, D., and Sjöqvist, F.:* Genetic control of nortriptyline kinetics in man. A study of relatives of propositi with high plasma concentrations. J. med. Genet. *8:* 129–135 (1971).
20 *Burrows, G.; Scoggins, B., and Davies, B.:* Plasma nortriptyline and clinical response. Presented at Symp. Media Hoechst Response to Treatment of Depression, Erbach 1973.
21 *Lehmann, M. and Silk, E.:* Familial pseudocholinesterase defficience. Brit. med. J. *i:* 128, 129 (1961).
22 *Winokur, G.; Morrison, J.; Clancy, J., and Crowe, R.:* Iowa 500. Clinical and genetic distinction of hebephrenic and paranoid schizophrenic. J. nerv. ment. Dis. *159:* 12–19 (1974).
23 *Tsuang, M. and Winokur, G.:* Criteria for subtyping process schizophrenia. I. Clinical differential of hebephrenic and paranoid schizophrenia. Arch. gen. Psychiat. *31:* 43–47 (1974).
24 *Kallmann, F.:* The genetics of schizophrenia (Augustin, New York 1938).
25 *Schulz, B.:* Zur Erbpathologie der Schizophrenie. Z. ges. Neurol. Psychiat. *143:* 175–293 (1932).
26 *Letemendia, F. and Harris, A.:* Chlorpromazine and the untreated chronic schizophrenic. A long term trial. Brit. J. Psychiat. *113:* 950–958 (1967).

Dr. *George Winokur*, MD, Department of Psychiatry, University of Iowa College of Medicine, *Iowa City, IA 52242* (USA)

Genetics and Psychopharmacology. Mod. Probl. Pharmacopsych., vol. 10, pp. 12–22, ed. *J. Mendlewicz*, Brussels (Karger, Basel 1975)

Alcoholism
A Pharmacogenetic Disorder

Gilbert S. Omenn

Division of Medical Genetics, University of Washington, Seattle, Wash.

I. Introduction

Alcoholism may be defined with clinical and pharmacological criteria as a behavioral disorder in which excessive drinking leads to tolerance, physical dependence, bodily injury and social opprobrium. For those interested in the biological bases of human behavior, alcoholism is a potentially fruitful research problem because the precipitating agent is well-known and because there are millions of affected individuals. Furthermore, evidence is accumulating that the predisposition to alcoholism is significantly influenced by inherited factors and that there are marked individual differences in the acute and chronic effects of ethanol.

The long-recognized higher incidence of alcoholism among family members of alcoholics, compared with the relatives of nonalcoholics (1), could be due to either inherited factors or the social environment or an interaction of both kinds of factors. Obviously, a higher familial incidence does not necessarily imply genetic determination. Nevertheless, despite the widespread assumption that the social effects on children of alcoholics were determinant, evidence has been put forth from new types of family studies that strongly point to genetic predisposition to alcoholism. These new types of studies employ half-siblings or adopted individuals, so that biologically related family members and nonbiologically related rearing family members can be compared. In this way, inherited and family environmental factors can be distinguished.

Schuckit (2) and *Schuckit et al.* (3) studied individuals reared apart from at least one of their biological parents in situations where either a biological parent or a 'surrogate' parent was diagnosed as an alcoholic. The half-sibling subjects were significantly more likely to have a drinking problem if their biological parent was considered alcoholic than if their surrogate (rearing) parent was alcoholic. Among 32 alcoholics and 132 nonalcoholics, most of whom came from broken homes, 62 % of the alcoholics had an alcoholic biological parent compared to 20 % of the nonalcoholics. This association occurred whether or not there had been physical contact with the alcoholic biological parent. Simply living with an alcoholic parent, on the other hand, appeared to have no relationship to the development of alcoholism.

Goodwin et al. (4) identified 55 men who had been separated from their biological parents in the first 6 weeks of life where one parent had a hospital diagnosis of alcoholism. Two control groups were matched for sex, age and time of adoption; one had no psychopathology in the parental histories, while the other control group represented families in which one parent had been hospitalized for a psychiatric condition other than alcoholism. The adoptees who had a biological parent with alcoholism (85 % of them the father) had a significantly higher incidence of alcoholism and hospitalization and psychiatric treatment for alcoholism. Except for a higher divorce rate, the alcoholic-offspring and control groups did not differ for anxiety neurosis, depression, sociopathy, drug addiction, heavy drinking without alcoholic features or any other variable studied. *Goodwin et al.* (5) have further analyzed their Danish sample for instances in which the adopted sons of alcoholics had a full brother raised by the biological alcoholic parent. In all, 35 such brothers were identified for 20 probands. The main finding was that sons of alcoholics were no more likely to become alcoholic if they were reared by their alcoholic parent than if they were separated from their alcoholic parent soon after birth and raised by nonrelatives. This finding held despite the fact that, as a group, the nonadoptees were older than their adopted brothers and presumably further into the age of risk for alcoholism, and despite the evidence that the nonadopted children had had a more disruptive social environment in childhood.

Beyond such impressive statistical evidence from family studies, we have noted (6) that there are several physiological and clinical levels at which genetic factors may be expected to play a role in the total picture of alcohol use and abuse (table I). The proverbial 'man in the street' likewise is certain to assert that there *are* striking differences between individuals in tolerance for alcohol and in susceptibility to its effects. The acute metabolic consequences of ethanol in the liver have been studied in considerable detail (7), but the metabolic nature of tolerance and cellular adaptation in the central nervous system (CNS) remains obscure (8). For both acute and chronic effects of excessive drinking there are

Table I. Levels of genetic influence in alcoholism

1. Susceptibility to acute intoxicating effects
2. Metabolism of ethanol
3. Central nervous system cellular adaptation to chronic intake – addictability
4. Predisposing personality factors
5. Susceptibility to medical and behavioral complications

still surprisingly few studies on the individual differences so intuitively perceived.

These results do not identify the particular genes involved in predisposition to alcoholism, nor do they identify any particular pattern of inheritance. It is quite likely that several independent mechanisms of genetically determined metabolic variations may predispose in different families to pharmacologic response and behavior that is diagnosed as alcoholism. This variety of mechanisms is termed 'genetic heterogeneity'.

A. Acute Effects of Ethanol

One remarkable difference among individuals, which appears to be distributed racially, is the striking facial flushing and increased pulse pressure observed promptly after ingestion of small amounts of alcohol by native Japanese, Taiwanese and Koreans. Ingestion of similar amounts of alcohol by American Caucasians usually has no detectable effect (9). The difference is not conditioned by experience, since *Wolff* was able to demonstrate the same difference in the neonatal period. Any quantitative association between intensity of flushing and habitual alcohol consumption could not be determined in Oriental populations because most Asian mongoloids and Amerasians abstain altogether from drinking alcohol. More recently, *Wolff* (10) has shown that North American Indians (Eastern Cree of the Algonquin family), anthropologically related to the Chinese and Japanese, have similar high incidence (80 %) and intensity of flushing after ingesting alcohol. In this group, heavy alcohol consumption could be shown to decrease somewhat the intensity of vasomotor response. The pharmacological mechanism responsible for the alcohol flushing and for the population differences observed is unknown. It is possible that a different metabolite or a larger fraction of one metabolite, such as acetaldehyde, is formed in Orientals and Indians, but there is so far no positive evidence to support such a speculation. Alternatively, there may be differences in the reactivity of the autonomic nervous system or its vascular supply of ethanol and its usual products.

In general, acute intoxicating effects are correlated with blood concentration of ethanol. Thus, the next level of investigation is the rate of metabolism of ethanol.

B. Metabolism of Ethanol

Studies of the rate of elimination of ethanol from the blood in monozygotic and dizygotic twins indicate that genetic factors are almost entirely responsible for individual differences; the heritability is estimated at 0.98 (11). Similar studies of antipyrine, phenylbutazone, bishydroxycoumarin and, to a lesser extent, halothane show that environmental contributions may be negligible compared with genetic factors in nonmedicated, nonhospitalized healthy twins. This extent of genetic control over the variation in drug metabolism has come as a surprise to many experimental pharmacologists familiar with the striking effects of dosage schedules, cage conditions, diet, etc.

Ethnic or racial differences in rate of metabolism of ethanol have been reported, as well. Casual police observations and lay impressions indicated that Eskimos and Indians in western Canada take longer to sober up after an alcoholic binge than do Caucasians in the same area (12). Differences in rate of metabolism of ethanol were shown to account for these observations. The amount of alcohol required per unit of body weight to induce or maintain an intoxicated state was similar in all 3 groups, but the rate of decline in blood alcohol levels was significantly lower in both the Eskimo and Indian groups than in the Caucasian.

In analyzing individual differences in rates of ethanol elimination from the blood, it is appropriate to ask which metabolic step or steps may determine these individual differences. Alcohol dehydrogenase (ADH) in the liver is generally thought to be the rate-limiting step for degradation of ethanol to acetaldehyde (which is converted further), though microsomal oxidizing systems play a part. A variant of ADH has been described in man by *von Wartburg and Schürch* (13) in 20 % of 59 liver specimens from a Swiss population and 4 % of 50 livers from an English sample. *Smith et al.* (14) have found this 'atypical' ADH in 10 % of a larger English sample (220 liver and lung specimens). The properties of the atypical ADH have been characterized with several techniques. A difference in the pH activity profile exists, so that the ratio of activity at pH 10.8 to that at pH 8.8 is greater than 1.0 for the normal enzyme and less than 1.0 for the atypical enzyme. A chelator of zinc in the ADH molecule, *o*-phenanthroline, inhibits the normal more than the atypical ADH, whereas the reverse is true for inhibition by pyrazol. In addition, there are differences in the relative rates with an array of substrates. ADH is not at all specific for ethanol. Most important, the total activity of the atypical enzyme is considerably higher than that of the normal enzyme in liver. Attempts were made to correlate, after intravenous infusion of ethanol, rates of degradation of the drug in patients whose ADH type had been determined from liver biopsies obtained at surgery (15). Two of their 23 subjects had atypical ADH: in the male subject with atypical ADH, capacity to metabolize ethanol (EtOH) was not different from that in males with typical ADH; in the female subject with atypical ADH, rate of EtOH degradation was greater than in a small group of females with typical ADH. To the present, the question of whether individuals with atypical ADH possess increased capacity to degrade ethanol and increased resistance to alcoholic cirrhosis remains unresolved. There appear to have been no studies of different racial groups (Eskimos,

Indians, Orientals) or of patients with cirrhosis for frequency of the atypical ADH.

Considerable progress has been made in characterizing the developmental and tissue-specific pattern of alcohol dehydrogenase isozymes (14, 16, 17). In early human fetal liver, there is a single band of ADH activity upon specific staining of starch gels after electrophoresis of liver homogenates. Additional bands of activity appear late in fetal life and also around adolescence (16). A switch in adolescence suggests a role for sex hormones. *Smith et al.* have elucidated the probable genetic control of ADH isozyme patterns in the liver and other tissues; one genetic locus directs synthesis of α-polypeptides in the fetus; later another locus (ADH$_2$) directs synthesis of β-polypeptides, leading to $\alpha\beta$ and $\beta\beta$ dimer enzyme molecules which can be distinguished electrophoretically. In the stomach and kidney and, to a lesser extent, in the liver, ADH$_3$ contributes yet another polypeptide, γ, with differing electrophoretic mobility. These electrophoretic studies seem to have elucidated also the origin of the atypical enzyme as a variant of the β-polypeptide and its ADH$_2$ gene. Since all these studies have been carried out with tissues obtained at autopsy, there has been no opportunity to confirm the genetic patterns with family data.

C. Tolerance and Physical Dependence

In man and in models of drinking behavior in animals, it is still not clear whether the active metabolic species in the nervous system is ethanol or acetaldehyde or some other product. Our understanding of the mechanisms and sites of metabolic impact of the agent is similarly limited for other tissues.

Tolerance, however, is susceptible to direct study in man. It should be possible to ascertain whether tolerance is mediated by faster degradation of the active species by the liver, so that lower concentrations reach the CNS, or whether similar or higher concentrations reach the CNS but find it less responsive. There is good evidence in man and animals that the CNS becomes adapted to higher concentrations of alcohol and opiates. *Goldstein and Sheehan* (18) have developed a promising model for morphine addiction in the mouse, in which quantifiable running fits decrease upon chronic exposure. Measurements of free, active drug have shown that high concentrations were present in the brains of tolerant mice (19). McClearn's model of fall time and sleep time in mice given intraperitoneal ethanol (20) may serve as a similar model for the tolerant or addicted state in alcoholism. If conditions were developed for nerve cell adaptation in tissue culture, careful comparison of the effects of EtOH and acetaldehyde could be carried out. Actual cellular receptors for addicting agents in alcoholism have yet to be identified. However, substantial progress has been reported in the characterization of opiate receptors in rat, monkey and human brain. Based upon the prediction of *Goldstein et al.* (21) that these receptors should be stereospecific, *Snyder* and his colleagues have employed radioactively labeled naloxone (22) and dihydromorphine (23) to demonstrate opiate receptors. Receptor sites are confined to nervous tissue and vary strikingly in number from region to region of brain, the richest regions belonging to the limbic system (23).

A chemical speculation has been advanced that might provide a common basis for addictability. *Davis and Walsh* (24) noted that acetaldehyde can condense with norepinephrine or serotonin to form Schiff bases and then undergo spontaneous rearrangement to tetrahydroisoquinolines or tetrahydropapaveraline, which are structures similar to plant alkaloids with high addictive potency. There is no experimental demonstration of this suggestion. However, there are claims that strains of rats obtained by selective breeding for susceptibility to opiate addiction manifest similar 'relapsing' behavior when offered alcohol after periods of drinking followed by abstinence (25). It would be of great interest if some common mechanism mediated addictability to several agents, though each agent might interact with different specific cell receptors to initiate the process. As an analogy, many polypeptide hormones interact with specific cell surface receptors and then activate the enzyme adenylcyclase and release cyclic adenosine monophosphate (AMP), a mediator for intracellular effects of all of these hormones (26). Another interesting feature of the development of tolerance is that inhibitors of RNA and protein synthesis, such as actinomycin D, puromycin, cycloheximide and 8-azaguanine, inhibit the development of tolerance to morphine without blocking the acute reaction in nontolerant mice (27). The same inhibitors have been used to explore the range of macromolecules that might be involved in information processing for general memory. Thus, drug tolerance may be a special case of 'memory' function.

D. Personality Factors

A great many studies have been performed to assess the personality profiles of alcoholics, though it is not always clear which features antedate the onset of alcoholism and which accompany or result from the excessive drinking behavior. Follow-up studies on large groups of individuals for whom personality batteries given during adolescence are available might reveal common personality factors that predispose to alcoholism, rather than reflect it. The relative roles of nature and nurture for many personality traits can be assessed by comparison of monozygotic twins reared together and monozygotic twins reared apart (28) and by comparison of biological and adoptive relatives of individuals who were adopted early in life or who are half-sibs. *Shields'* data suggest a significant heritability for a number of traits of temperament.

E. Medical Complications of Alcoholism

1. Cirrhosis

Internists who see the medical complications of alcoholism find that only about 5–10 % of alcoholics with similar long histories of abuse of alcohol and inadequate diet develop cirrhosis of the liver. A similarly small percentage develops recurrent pancreatitis. The biochemical or metabolic characteristics of the liver or pancreas that determine susceptibility to deleterious effects of excessive EtOH ingestion are not known. One curious observation that might be relevant is that individuals with cirrhosis lack the normal amount of body hair. *Chvostek* several decades ago (29) and *Muller* 20 years ago (30) documented hypotrichosis as a premorbid feature of men who develop cirrhosis. Table II gives the different distribution of hairiness in a control population and in a group of cirrhotics.

This point is mentioned for two reasons. First, subgroups of alcoholics at special risk for cirrhosis or other complications of chronic alcoholism might be identified by relatively simple clinical criteria, as well as by biochemical features. Second, there may be a hormonal basis for the difference in body-hair distribution that serves as a clue to biochemical mechanisms. Testosterone does induce ADH activity in mouse kidney, but not in mouse liver (31). It is not known whether ADH is inducible in man by testosterone or which of the many other enzymes induced by androgenic hormones in man might be important in withstanding the effects of alcoholism. It is possible that testosterone influences the maturational change reported at puberty for liver ADH isozymes (16).

Individuals with particular metabolic abnormalities may be unduly susceptible to exacerbation of that abnormality upon ingestion of ethanol. For example, subjects with hypertriglyceridemia have been shown to have a striking increase in fasting serum triglyceride levels upon moderate ethanol ingestion for 7 days, while subjects with normal blood lipids had no significant change in fasting plasma triglyceride levels on the same regimen (32).

2. Chronic Brain Syndromes

Differences among alcoholics in susceptibility to such complications as cerebellar degeneration or Korsakoff's confabulatory psychosis or deterioration of intellectual function may reflect differences in response to the direct effects of ethanol or to the associated or secondary nutritional deficiencies. Alcoholics may even differ in their risk of developing the thiamine-responsive Wernicke's encephalopathy if they have genetically determined differences in carbohydrate metabolism and in demand for thiamine. The possibility was raised above that analogous genetically determined differences in metabolic pathways in the liver may make individuals more or less susceptible to toxic effects of alcohol and dietary inadequacies.

We have applied techniques of electrophoretic screening for enzyme variants

Table II. Body-hair distribution and susceptibility to cirrhosis[1]

Hairiness class	Description	49 males with cirrhosis of the liver, %	500 normal males, %
I	no chest hair, little arm hair	85.8	20.4
II	moderate chest hair	12.2	71.8
III	much chest hair, down over abdomen to pubic hair	2.0	7.6

1 Age-matched males (30).

among a series of 150 human brain specimens. No common variants were identified for any of the 11 enzymes of the glycolytic pathway, the crucial metabolic process for energy metabolism (33). Among another dozen enzymes important to energy production and lipid biosynthesis, common variant forms were noted for glucose-6-phosphate dehydrogenase and 6-phosphogluconate dehydrogenase of the pentose-phosphate shunt pathway (variants already known to occur in the blood) and a remarkably high-frequency polymorphism for the mitochondrial malic enzyme [triphosphopyridine nucleotide (NADP)-linked malate dehydrogenase] was discovered (34). Such *in vitro* differences, when observed, must be related to physiological effects and, subsequently, to behavioral parameters or clinical complications. We are also using certain pharmacologic agents that act as enzyme inhibitors. Some of these inhibitors are being used clinically and many have been tested in animals for behavioral effects. Nearly every enzyme in the pathways of biosynthesis and degradation of the neurotransmitters norepinephrine, serotonin, acetylcholine and γ-aminobutyric acid can be tested for individual differences in the extent of inhibition by specific inhibitors. This work is at an early stage and requires tissue samples, but carries the promise of leading to a 'genetic profile' of metabolic pathways that might underlie hereditary predisposition to common diseases.

No simple, mendelian single-gene hypothesis will account for the complex and surely heterogeneous phenotype we recognize as alcoholism. The drug, ethanol, is essential of course to the development of the signs of this pharmacogenetic disorder. It seems likely that individuals do differ in their genes for key enzymes in the liver and in the brain, thereby having differences in addictability of nerve cells, and differing personality traits. Hopefully, more sophisticated understanding of the biological and psychological bases of predisposition to alcoholism will point the way to more effective and more specific measures of therapy and prevention.

3. Fetal Alcohol Syndrome

Among children born to mothers who were chronic alcoholics, a striking new malformation syndrome has been recognized (35). These children have retarded intrauterine and postnatal physical and mental development, microcephaly, decreased width to the palpebral fissure causing the eyes to appear rounded, and variable limb and cardiac malformations. The degree of linear growth deficiency was more severe than the deficit of weight at birth, which is quite uncommon. The mechanism of toxicity and the issue of genetic variation in susceptibility are not yet resolved. However, the original report of 8 cases included Caucasian, Negro and American Indian children. Subsequently, *Jones and Smith* (36) have presented autopsy findings in one case, distinguished by aberrant neuronal migration in the brain, a family with 2 children affected, and another family in which a woman had 7 normal children before she became alcoholic and then had 3 spontaneous abortions and an affected child after she was alcoholic. Likely occurrences of this syndrome were identified in Greek and Roman myths and in British reports of a century ago. *Jones et al.* (37) also have reviewed the data of the large Collaborative Study on Perinatal Morbidity in a search for additional cases. Among the offspring of 23 women identified as chronic alcoholics, 4 died in the perinatal period, 6 had the features of this fetal alcohol syndrome and others had less severe growth retardation and intellectual impairment at age 7 years.

Summary

Alcoholism is an extremely common psychosocial behavioral disorder for which genetic factors may play an important role. Statistical analysis of special kinds of family studies that separate inherited factors from the common family environment point strongly to genetic predisposition. This paper presents data and speculations on the genetically determined differences among population subgroups and individuals in the acute effects of ethanol ingestion, the metabolism of ethanol, the process of tolerance, physical dependence and addictability, premorbid personality features and serious complications of alcoholism in the liver and brain of the alcoholic and in the offspring of alcoholic mothers.

References

1   *Winokur, G.; Reich, I.; Rimmer, J., and Pitts, F.N., jr.:* Alcoholism. III. Diagnosis and familial psychiatric illness in 259 alcoholic probands. Arch. gen. Psychiat. *23:* 104–111 (1970).
2   *Schuckit, M.A.:* Family history and half-sibling research in alcoholism. In Nature and Nurture in Alcoholism. Ann. N.Y. Acad. Sci. *197:* 121–124 (1972).

3 *Schuckit, M.A.; Goodwin, D.W., and Winokur, G.:* A study of alcoholism in half siblings. Amer. J. Psychiat. *128:* 122–126 (1972).

4 *Goodwin, D.W.; Schulsinger, F.; Hermansen, L.; Guze, S.B., and Winokur, G.:* Alcohol problems in adoptees raised apart from alcoholic biological parents. Arch. gen. Psychiat. *28:* 238–243 (1973).

5 *Goodwin, D.W.; Schulsinger, F.; Moller, N.; Hermansen, L.; Winokur, G., and Guze, S.B.:* Drinking problems in adopted and nonadopted sons of alcoholics. Arch. gen. Psychiat. *31:* 164–169 (1974).

6 *Omenn, G.S. and Motulsky, A.G.:* A biochemical and genetic approach to alcoholism. Ann. N.Y. Acad. Sci. *197:* 16–23 (1972).

7 *Lieber, C.S.:* Liver adaptation and injury in alcoholism. New Engl. J. Med. *288:* 356–362 (1973).

8 *Mendelson, J.H.:* Biologic concomitants of alcoholism. New Engl. J. Med. *283:* 71–81 (1970).

9 *Wolff, P.H.:* Ethnic differences in alcohol sensitivity. Science *175:* 449–450 (1972).

10 *Wolff, P.H.:* Vasomotor sensitivity to alcohol in diverse mongoloid populations. Amer. J. hum. Genet. *25:* 193–199 (1973).

11 *Vesell, E.S.; Page, J.G., and Passananti, G.T.:* Genetic and environmental factors affecting ethanol metabolism in man. Clin. Pharmacol. Ther. *12:* 192–201 (1971).

12 *Fenna, D.; Mix, L.; Schaefer, O., and Gilbert, J.A.L.:* Ethanol metabolism in various racial groups. Canad. med. Ass. J. *105:* 472–475 (1971).

13 *Wartburg, J.P. von and Schürch, P.M.:* Atypical human liver alcohol dehydrogenase. Ann. N.Y. Acad. Sci. *151:* 936–947 (1968).

14 *Smith, M.; Hopkinson, D.A., and Harris, H.:* Developmental changes and polymorphism in human alcohol dehydrogenase. Ann. hum. Genet., Lond. *34:* 251–271 (1971).

15 *Edwards, J.A. and Price Evans, D.A.:* Ethanol metabolism in subjects possessing typical and atypical liver alcohol dehydrogenase. Clin. Pharmacol. Ther. *8:* 824–829 (1967).

16 *Murray, R.F., jr. and Motulsky, A.G.:* Developmental variation in the isoenzymes of human liver and gastric alcohol dehydrogenase. Science *171:* 71–72 (1971).

17 *Smith, M.; Hopkinson, D.A., and Harris, H.:* Studies on the properties of the human alcohol dehydrogenase isozymes determined by the different loci ADH_1, ADH_2, ADH_3. Ann. hum. Genet., Lond. *37:* 49–67 (1973).

18 *Goldstein, A. and Sheehan, P.:* Tolerance to opiate narcotics. I. Tolerance to the 'running fit' caused by levorphanol in the mouse. J. Pharmacol. exp. Ther. *169:* 175 (1969).

19 *Richter, J.A. and Goldstein, A.:* Tolerance to opiate narcotics. II. Cellular tolerance to levorphanol in mouse brain. Proc. nat. Acad. Sci., Wash. *66:* 944–951 (1970).

20 *Kakihana, R.; Brown, D.R.; McClearn, G.E., and Tabershaw, I.R.:* Brain sensitivity to alcohol in inbred mouse strains. Science *154:* 1574–1575 (1966).

21 *Goldstein, A.; Lowney, L.E., and Pal, B.K.:* Stereospecific and nonspecific interactions of the morphine congener levophanol in subcellular fractions of mouse brain. Proc. nat. Acad. Sci., Wash. *68:* 1742–1747 (1971).

22 *Pert, C.B. and Snyder, S.H.:* Properties of opiate-receptor binding in rat brain. Proc. nat. Acad. Sci., Wash. *70:* 2243–2247 (1973).

23 *Kuhar, M.J.; Pert, C.B., and Snyder, S.H.:* Regional distribution of opiate receptor binding in monkey and human brain. Nature, Lond. *245:* 447–450 (1973).

24 *Davis, V.E. and Walsh, M.J.:* Alcohol, amines, alkaloids. A possible biochemical basis for alcohol addiction. Science *167:* 1005–1007 (1970).

25 *Nichols, J.R. and Hsaio, S.:* Addiction liability of albino rats. Breeding for quantitative differences in morphine drinking. Science *157:* 561–563 (1967).

26 *Sutherland, E.W.:* On the biologic role of cyclic AMP. J. amer. med. Ass. *214:* 1281–1288 (1970).
27 *Way, E.L.; Loh, H.D., and Shen, F.H.:* Morphine tolerance, physical dependence and synthesis of brain 5-hydroxytryptamine. Science *162:* 1290–1292 (1968).
28 *Shields, J.:* Monozygotic twins brought up apart and brought up together (Oxford Univ. Press, New York 1962).
29 *Chvostek, F.:* Klinische Vorträge. Zur Pathogenese der Leberzirrhose. Wiener klin. Wschr. *35:* 381 (1922).
30 *Muller, G.:* Der erbkonstitutionelle Hypogenitalismus des Mannes als Dispositions-faktor der Lebercirrhose. Med. Klin. *71* (1952).
31 *Ohno, S.; Stenius, C., and Christian, L.C.:* Sex difference in alcohol metabolism. Androgenic steroid as an inducer of kidney alcohol dehydrogenase. Clin. Genet. *1:* 35 (1970).
32 *Ginsberg, H.; Olefsky, J.; Farquhar, J.W., and Reaven, G.M.:* Moderate ethanol ingestion and plasma triglyceride levels. A study in normal and hypertriglyceridemic persons. Ann. intern. Med. *80:* 143–149 (1974).
33 *Cohen, P.T.W.; Omenn, G.S.; Motulsky, A.G.; Chen, S.H., and Giblett, E.R.:* Restricted variation in the glycolytic enzymes of human brain and erythrocytes. Nature, Lond. *241:* 229–233 (1973).
34 *Cohen, P.T.W. and Omenn, G.S.:* Human malic enzyme. High frequency polymorphism of the mitochondrial form. Biochem. Genet. *7:* 303–311 (1972).
35 *Jones, K.K.; Smith, D.W.; Ulleland, C.N., and Streissguth, A.P.:* Pattern of malformation in offspring of chronic alcoholic mothers. Lancet *i:* 1267–1271 (1973).
36 *Jones, K.L. and Smith, D.W.:* Recognition of the fetal alcohol syndrome in early infancy. Lancet *ii:* 999–1001 (1973).
37 *Jones, K.L.; Smith, D.W.; Streissguth, A.P., and Myrianthopoulos, N.C.:* Outcome in offspring of chronic alcoholic women. Lancet *i:* 1076–1078 (1974).

Dr. *Gilbert S. Omenn,* MD, PhD, Associate Professor of Medicine, University of Seattle, *Seattle, WA 98195* (USA)

Genetics and Psychopharmacology. Mod. Probl. Pharmacopsych., vol. 10, pp. 23–29,
ed. *J. Mendlewicz,* Brussels (Karger, Basel 1975)

Genetic Factors and Lithium Response in Manic-Depressive Illness

J. Mendlewicz and F. Stallone

Department of Medical Genetics and Department of Internal Medicine, New York
State Psychiatric Institute, and Department of Psychiatry, Columbia University, New
York, N.Y.

Introduction

Individual differences in handling drugs have been well documented in many
pharmacological studies both in animals and humans. Several investigators have
recently shown that drug metabolism and, thus, drug response as well as side-
effects of these drugs are often the result of a complex interaction between
genetic and environmental factors. Pharmacogenetics, which was originally
limited to the description of clinical syndromes induced by hereditary variation
in the handling of certain drugs, is now being extended to the study of polymorphic systems in man (such as the pseudocholinesterase polymorphism) and
also to the therapy of genetic syndromes. Several examples of the influence of
genetic factors in neuropsychopharmacology have recently been described. The
isoniazid acetyltransferase polymorphism is one of them and may account for
differences in therapeutic response to phenelzine in depressed patients (*Johnstone and Marsh,* 1973). Plasma levels of diphenylhydantoin, phenobarbital and
nortriptyline (used in the treatment of both neurological and psychiatric diseases) also appear to be genetically determined (*Åsberg et al.,* 1971; *Kutt,* 1971;
Vesell, 1973). These observations are of great importance, since clinical response
to these psychoactive drugs has been shown to be related to their plasma levels.

One of the most remarkable drugs available in psychiatry today is the
lithium salts. When lithium is administered chronically to affectively ill patients,
it prevents a recurrence of future episodes of mania and possibly depression. The
long-term stabilizing properties of lithium in bipolar manic-depressive illness
have been found in various controlled longitudinal studies recently reviewed by
Prien et al. (1974). Although the time periods during which the patients were
studied are not always similar in the various studies, and although control procedures are not always as stringent as they should be, the long-term prophylactic

response of bipolar manic-depressive patients treated with lithium is significantly superior to that of control patients treated with a placebo.

However, failures on lithium maintenance do occur, an observation that has aroused considerable speculation. Certain methodological artifacts may in some cases account for lithium failures. For instance, so-called 'failures' may be patients who were misdiagnosed as manic-depressive, but actually had a schizophrenic, neurotic or some other disorder which is known not to respond to lithium treatment. Further, long-term lithium treatment also requires periodic evaluation of plasma lithium levels. To obtain a full tissue effect, the serum lithium level should be maintained between 0.9 and 1.2 mEq/l. This is a rough estimate, because it may vary with age, weight, thyroid function and other variables as yet unknown. Plasma levels below 0.8 mEq/l would indicate that lithium dosage is insufficient and may account for the recurrence of an affective episode. Thus, some 'failures' might be the result of inadequate drug dosages.

Aside from the methodological artifacts that might account for failures of lithium prophylaxis, there exists an alternative explanation that has important theoretical implications: there may be significant differences between patients in the handling of this drug. Several studies point to this possibility. A recent study reported by *Serry* (1969) points to differences in the metabolism of lithium among patients with affective disorders. This investigator has studied the urinary excretion of lithium by affectively ill patients. This was done by administrating to these patients a loading dose of lithium carbonate during mania. Patients who were found to be slow urinary excretors tended to respond favorably to lithium treatment, while patients who were rapid excretors tended not to respond to the drug. *Cade* (1970) has also shown that lithium excretion might be a predicting factor in the rate of lithium response. However, other investigators (*Stokes et al.*, 1972) were not able to confirm these interesting results.

Another possibility which should be taken into account in the differential response rate of manic-depressive patients is the possibility that this disease encompasses several biologically different syndromes, some of which may be lithium-responsive and others lithium-resistant. The isolation of a group of patients with affective disorders who do not respond to lithium, perhaps for biological reasons, raises the further possibility that manic-depressive patients who are lithium nonresponders might be genetically different from those who are lithium responders. There is mounting evidence from both clinical and genetic studies for the heterogenic nature of manic-depressive illness (*Mendlewicz et al.*, 1972; *Mendlewicz et al.*, 1973a; *Mendlewicz*, 1974). The investigation of familial genetic factors as they relate to treatment response in manic-depressive patients may further clarify the definition of the subtypes of this disorder.

We have previously presented data suggesting a relationship between a patient's response to long-term lithium treatment and his genetic background (*Mendlewicz et al.*, 1973b). *Prien et al.* (1974), studying factors associated with treatment success in lithium prophylaxis, have recently published results suggesting such an association. The present study extends our preliminary investigations to a larger sample of patients in order to further test the above hypothesis.

Sample and Methods

All patients consecutively admitted in a double-blind study of lithium prophylaxis for bipolar illness were identified as probands for the purpose of doing family studies. All the available first-degree relatives and spouses of the probands were personally examined with scales designed to measure both current and past psychopathology (*Endicott and Spitzer*, 1972) in order to assess the prevalence of psychopathology in these families. These studies were part of overall family studies of affectively ill patients, some of whom were included in the lithium prophylactic studies. The criteria for diagnosing bipolar illness in probands and relatives were a history of clear-cut manic episodes and depressive episodes serious enough to require treatment or to cause a disruption in everyday activities for at least 3 weeks. Periodicity of the illness with free intervals was among the criteria used for diagnosing bipolar illness. Unipolar illness was diagnosed in individuals who had never been manic or hypomanic, but had experienced one or more depressive episodes severe enough to require treatment or to cause a disruption in normal social functioning for at least 3 weeks. Patients evidencing personality disintegration before or after a psychotic episode, or having other pre-existing psychiatric or medical disease that might be associated with an affective symptomatology, were not diagnosed as affectively ill patients. These diagnostic criteria are similar to the concept of primary affective disorder proposed by *Robins and Guze* (1972). The evaluation of lithium prophylaxis in this study requires a patient to be normothymic at randomination and to be followed for at least 6 months. The investigator interviewing relatives was blind to which probands were treated with lithium or placebo and to the proband's treatment response. The methods used to conduct the family history studies have been described previously (*Mendlewicz et al.*, 1972). The research plan of the double-blind study was started in October, 1969, and the study is still in progress today. Data up to 48 months were analyzed for this study. 43 bipolar patients were assigned to lithium carbonate on a random basis and 46 to placebo. Plasma lithium levels were monitored once every 4 weeks, and dosage was adjusted to maintain a serum lithium level between 0.8 and 1.3 mEq/l. All patients taking placebo were given a fictitious lithium plasma level to help maintain the blindness of the study. If a patient was considered by at least 2 separate blind evaluators to be ill enough to require additional medication (other than lithium) or hospitalization for an acute episode, he was considered a lithium failure. Details on the methods and preliminary results of this double-blind study of lithium prophylaxis have been published elsewhere (*Stallone et al.*, 1973).

Results

Table I summarizes the clinical results on 89 bipolar manic-depressive patients randomly assigned to lithium (43) and placebo (46) and who were followed up to 48 months. Of the 43 bipolar patients followed on lithium carbonate, 24 (56 %) were long-term responders and 19 (44 %) were long-term

Table I. Response to lithium or placebo in 89 manic-depressive patients

	Lithium patients	Placebo patients
Responders	24	13
Nonresponders	19	33
Total	43	46

failures. The lithium plasma levels for both the responders and the failures were regularly maintained between 0.8 and 1.3 mEq/l. In a previous report (*Mendlewicz et al.*, 1973b) based on a double-blind study of 36 bipolar patients on lithium followed-up for a shorter period (37 months), 67 % were responders and 33 % were long-term failures. This seems to indicate that the response rate lessens as the follow-up period on lithium maintenance therapy is prolonged. Ultimately, perhaps, if patients are followed for a sufficiently long period even the most responsive to lithium may develop episodes. Of the 46 bipolar patients followed on placebo, in the present study 13 (28 %) were responders and 33 (72 %) were long-term failures. Thus, bipolar patients on placebo for up to 48 months do significantly worse than bipolar patients on lithium for the same study period ($\chi^2 = 6.93$, df = 1, p < 0.01). In contrast to the lithium group, the placebo group shows a slightly better response rate than the one obtained in our previous study (*Mendlewicz et al.*, 1973b) in which 36 bipolar patients were followed on placebo for 37 months. Of these, 25 % were responders and 75 % were long-term failures. It is noteworthy that 28 % of bipolar patients on placebo do not present any relapse after being followed for up to 48 months.

The present study is aimed at comparing the genetic background of bipolar patients on lithium and placebo in reference to long-term clinical response. Four samples of patients are thus available for our analysis: responders and failures treated with lithium and responders and failures under placebo. The mean number of first-degree relatives who were alive is similar in all 4 samples (range: 4.5–5.3/family). The mean number of relatives interviewed was also similar (range: 3.5–4.5/family). The age distribution of first-degree relatives in the lithium and placebo groups were comparable. Table II gives the incidence of responders and nonresponders to lithium with respect to the presence or absence of bipolar and unipolar illness in the proband's first-degree relatives: 16 of 24 responders to lithium had a positive family history of bipolar illness while only 4 of the 19 nonresponders had a positive family history of bipolar illness ($\chi^2 = 7.14$, df = 1, p < 0.01)[1] for small numbers was used in all analysis. However, 17 lithium responders had a positive family history of unipolar illness, compared with 12 patients in the nonresponder group ($\chi^2 = 0.04$, d.f. = 1, not significant

1   χ^2 with Yates correction for small numbers was used in all analyses.

Table II. Incidence of affective illness in first-degree relatives of responder and nonresponder manic-depressive patients

Affective illness in family	Lithium patients			Placebo patients		
	responders	nonresponders	total	responders	nonresponders	total
Bipolar illness	16	4	20	4	17	21
No bipolar illness	8	15	23	9	16	25
Total	24	19	43	13	33	46
Unipolar illness	17	12	29	8	23	31
No unipolar illness	7	7	14	5	10	15
Total	24	19	43	13	33	46

[NS]). The significant association found between family history of bipolar illness and long-term lithium response may also reflect a lower frequency of affective episodes in bipolar patients with a positive family history of the illness, irrespective of lithium treatment. The association was, therefore, examined separately for the placebo group. Table II shows an absence of any association between history of either bipolar or unipolar illness and 'long-term response' to placebo ($\chi^2 = 0.88$, d.f. = 1, NS for bipolar illness; $\chi^2 = 0.12$ d.f. = 1, NS for unipolar illness).

Discussion

The clinical findings in this study clearly demonstrate the superiority of lithium carbonate over placebo in preventing affective episodes in bipolar manic-depressive patients followed in a prospective study of lithium prophylaxis. However, the long-term response of bipolar patients treated with lithium is not as impressive, since only 56 % show an unequivocal prophylaxis (for both mania and depression) after being followed for 48 months. The isolation of a significant group of bipolar patients (44 %) who do not respond to lithium prophylaxis in a 4-year study, raises the question as to whether long-term lithium failures are clinically or genetically different from long-term lithium responders. It has been suggested (*Mendlewicz et al.*, 1973c) that previously treated lithium patients who have managed to adhere to a lithium regimen in an outpatient clinic: i.e. 'old cases', are more likely to respond to lithium treatment than do 'new cases', never treated with lithium before. Patients who experience more affective episodes during a short time period also seem to be less manageable on long-term lithium treatment (*Prien et al.*, 1974). It is unclear whether these clinical differences have any biological implications. Our finding that lithium prophylaxis is related to the presence of mania in the family confirms and extends previous studies (*Mendlewicz et al.,* 1973 b; *Prien et al.,* 1974). Bipolar patients who are long-term lithium responders have, thus, a much greater chance to have other relatives affected with the same disease, i.e. bipolar illness. There seems to be no relationship, however, between long-term lithium response and the presence of unipolar illness only in the family. Furthermore, the prophylactic response to lithium is not restricted to those bipolar patients who have a positive family history of mania. Indeed, 8 patients who do not have bipolar illness in their first-degree relatives show long-term lithium response. The association found between treatment response and family history may point to genetic differences between lithium responders and lithium failures. However, environmental factors related to the presence of the same disease in the families of bipolar patients may also play a role in determining their long-range treatment response. For example, patients whose relatives have also experienced mania may be more aware of the social consequences of this disease, thus more prone to adhere to a continuous lithium regimen. Our results indicate that it is possible to isolate 2 subgroups of bipolar manic-depressive patients according to their lithium response, and that the 2 subgroups of the illness can also be isolated on the basis of clinical features (*Mendlewicz et al.,* 1972) and genetic analysis (*Mendlewicz et al.,* 1973 a). These findings indicate that genetic heterogeneity may be present in bipolar manic-depressive illness (*Mendlewicz,* 1974).

Summary

The relationship between success in lithium treatment and the presence of affective illness in the families of manic-depressive patients was investigated in a double-blind study of lithium prophylaxis. Of a total of 89 outpatients who were followed for periods of up to 48 months, 43 were randomly assigned to lithium and 46 to placebo. 56 % of the lithium-treated patients remained asymptomatic, as compared to 28 % of the placebo patients.

Of the 24 successfully treated lithium cases, 16 (66 %) had at least one first-degree relative with bipolar illness, while only 4 of the 19 lithium failures (21 %) had a first-degree relative with bipolar illness. No relationship was found between response to lithium and the presence of unipolar illness in the patients' families.

Acknowledgements

This work was supported by the Belgian-American Educational Foundation and by General Research Support Grant No. 303-E-165F to the New York State Psychiatric Institute.

The authors wish to express their gratitude to Dr. *R.R. Fieve* and Dr. *J.D. Rainer* for administratively facilitating the research. Acknowledgements are also due to *M. Cataldo* for her able research assistance.

References

Åsberg, M.; Price Evans, D.A., and Sjöqvist, F.: Genetic control of nortriptyline kinetics in man. A study of relatives of proposita with high plasma concentrations. J. med. Genet. *8:* 129–135 (1971).

Cade, J.F.J.: Lithium. Historical perspectives and present status (abstract); in Scientific proceedings in summary form. The 123rd Ann. Meeting of the APA, San Francisco 1970, p. 155 (American Psychiatric Association, Washington 1970).

Endicott, J. and Spitzer, R.L.: Current and past psychopathology scales. Rationale, reliability, and validity. Arch. gen. Psychiat. *27:* 678–687 (1972).

Johnstone, E.C. and Marsh, W.: Acetylator status and response to phenelzine in depressed patients. Lancet *i:* 567–570 (1973).

Kutt, H.: Biochemical and genetic factors regulating dilantin metabolism in man. Ann. N.Y. Acad. Sci. *179:* 704–722 (1971).

Mendlewicz, J.: Le concept d'hétérogénéité dans la psychose maniaco-dépressive. Implications génétiques et thérapeutiques. Inform. psychiat. *2:* 411–416 (1974).

Mendlewicz, J.; Fieve, R.R.; Rainer, J.D., and Cataldo, M.: Affective disorder on paternal and maternal sides. Observations in bipolar (manic-depressive) patients with and without a family history. Brit. J. Psychiat. *122:* 31–34 (1973a).

Mendlewicz, J.; Fieve, R.R.; Rainer, J.D., and Fleiss, J.L.: Manic-depressive illness. A comparative study of patients with and without a family history. Brit. J. Psychiat. *120:* 523–530 (1972).

Mendlewicz, J.; Fieve, R.R., and Stallone, F.: Relationship between the effectiveness of lithium therapy and family history. Amer. J. Psychiat. *130:* 1011–1013 (1973b).

Mendlewicz, J.; Fieve, R.R., and Stallone, F.: Genetic aspects of lithium prophylaxis in bipolar manic-depressive illness; in Ban Psychopharmacology, sexual disorders and drug abuse, pp. 309–317 (North-Holland, Amsterdam 1973c).

Prien, R.F.; Caffey, E.M., and Klett, C.J.: Factors associated with treatment success in lithium carbonate prophylaxis. Arch. gen. Psychiat. *31:* 189–192 (1974).

Robins, E. and Guze, S.B.: Classification of affective disorders. The primary-secondary, the endogenous-reactive, and the neurotic-psychotic concepts; in *Williams* Recent advances in the psychobiology of the depressive illness. DHEW Publication (HSM) 70-9053 (NIMH 1972).

Serry, M.: Lithium retention and response. Lancet *i:* 1267–1268 (1969).

Stallone, F.; Shelley, E.; Mendlewicz, J., and Fieve, R.: The use of lithium in affective disorders. III. A double-blind study of prophylaxis in bipolar illness. Amer. J. Psychiat. *130:* 1006–1010 (1973).

Stokes, J.W.; Mendels, J.; Secunda, S.K., and Dyson, W.L.: Lithium excretion and therapeutic response. J. nerv. ment. Dis. *154:* 43–48 (1972).

Vesell, E.S.: Advances in pharmacogenetics. Progr. med. Genet. *9:* 291–367 (1973).

Dr. *J. Mendlewicz*, Institut de Psychiatrie, ULB Hôpital Brugmann, 4 Place Van Gehuchten, *Bruxelles 1020* (Belgium)

Genetics and Psychopharmacology. Mod. Probl. Pharmacopsych., vol. 10, pp. 30–37,
ed. *J. Mendlewicz*, Brussels (Karger, Basel 1975)

Relationship between Acetylator Status and Response to Phenelzine

Eve C. Johnstone

Department of Psychological Medicine, University of Glasgow, Glasgow

In clinical practice it is an everyday observation that the response of patients to standard dosages of drugs is extremely variable. When a drug is administered in controlled conditions to large numbers of patients and a graph drawn of their response, a unimodal curve representing continuous variation may be found, but in some instances the curve will be bimodal or even trimodal, representing discontinuous variation.

It has, in the past, tended to be assumed that the variability of drug metabolism and response is of the unimodal continuous type (viz., in the individual patient, therapeutic or side-effects known to result from a given drug could be produced given adequate dosage) but there are examples of discontinuous variability which are of clinical relevance. Bimodal or trimodal distribution of response may represent two or three genetically determined phenotypes. The term 'polymorphism' is used when several phenotypes exist within the same population and are maintained from one generation to the next by genetic mechanisms. It is now known that there is a polymorphism for the acetylation of certain drugs.

Acetylation polymorphism was first studied with reference to the antituberculous drug isoniazid, which was shown to be effective in the treatment of tuberculosis in 1952 (1). Shortly afterwards it was found that patients differed greatly in the way in which they metabolised isoniazid (2). *Hughes et al.* showed that isoniazid was excreted as unchanged drug, as acetylated derivative and as other metabolites and that while the percentage of acetylated derivative varied among different subjects from 14 to 70 %, the pattern of excretion for the individual was constant. This and other studies suggested that the variability in the inactivation of isoniazid is of the discontinuous kind, i.e. that the population is divided into two classes, rapid and slow inactivators. Twin studies and racial studies (3, 4) suggested that there was a genetic basis for this polymorphism and the detailed study of 484 subjects by *Evans et al.* (5) offered definite evidence that this was the case. Intestinal absorption, protein binding, renal glomerular clearance and renal tubular absorption were found to be irrelevant to the polymorphism (6) and it seemed likely that the difference between the rapid and slow inactivators was metabolic. The fact that the proportion of free unchanged drug excreted varied inversely with the proportion of acetylated drug (2) tended to suggest that the difference lay in speed of acetylation. This idea was confirmed by *Evans and White* (7) who showed that the livers of rapid inactivators of isoniazid have greater acetylating powers than those of slow inactivators, and by *Peters et al.* (8) who showed that acetylation was the primary metabolic reaction determining inactivator status for isoniazid.

Satisfactory evidence was then available to show that the metabolism of isoniazid was determined by a genetic polymorphism controlling acetylation. The practical relevance of this was shown by studies indicating that slow inactivators of isoniazid had a greater liability than fast to develop isoniazid-induced peripheral neuropathy (10, 11). Clearly, it was likely that any drug metabolised by acetylation would be subject to this polymorphism and therefore the effects of such a drug in a random population would vary as a result. In fact, acetylation polymorphism accounts for little of the widespread variability in the response of human subjects to the vast range of drugs which they ingest, as few drugs are metabolised by this mechanism. Sulphadimidine is polymorphically acetylated (9) and there is evidence to suggest that hydrallazine (7, 12). and the hydrazine drug, phthivazid (13), are substrates for polymorphic acetylation. It is probable that derivatives of hydrazine would be metabolised in a similar way.

The anti-depressant drug, phenelzine, is a substituted hydrazine. This drug is a monoamine oxidase inhibitor (MAOI). Drugs of this group prevent the intra-neuronal deamination of monoamines and increase their concentration in the brain in both animals (14) and man (15). The fact that these drugs are effective in relieving depression is one of the pieces of evidence for the theory that monoamines have a central role in the aetiology of depressive illness. The poor response of some depressed patients (16) to these drugs has been disappointing from the point of view of management of the individual and from the point of view of the theory. *Pare et al.* (17) studied the response of depressed patients to anti-depressants of the MAOI group and of the tricyclic group to examine the responses of individual patients in succeeding illnesses and to compare the responses of first-degree relatives to these drugs. Patients tended to respond in a consistent way in succeeding illnesses and the responses of first-degree relatives were also consistent, suggesting that genetic factors might be of relevance.

Being a hydrazine derivative, phenelzine is likely to be subject to polymorphic acetylation. If this were so it would account for the variable results produced by the drug and for the apparent genetic tendency of the response. The possibility that the response of depressed patients to phenelzine might be related to acetylator status was studied in 1965 by *Evans et al.* (18). They

Table I. Details of patients studied at outset of project of *Evans et al.* (18)

Clinical classification	Rapid acetylators			Slow acetylators		
	number	age (years) and mean ± SEM	weight (kg) and mean ± SEM	number	age (years) and mean ± SEM	weight (kg) and mean ± SEM
Neurotic depression	9	35.11 ± 4.20	133.00 ± 9.95	16	38.44 ± 2.84	142.33 ± 6.53
Endogenous depression	8	38.38 ± 3.47	145.50 ± 11.19	17	48.59 ± 2.87	155.59 ± 7.14
Total	17	36.65 ± 2.70	138.88 ± 7.38	33	43.36 ± 2.36	149.37 ± 5.04

No significant differences in weight between slow and rapid acetylators.
Slow acetylators with endogenous depression have a higher mean age than the other three phenotypic and disease categories (p < 0.001).
Reproduced by kind permission of Prof. *D.A. Price Evans*, Liverpool.

Table II. Clinical responses observed (mean ± SEM of the ratios of each parameter before and after phenelzine therapy) in study of *Evans et al.* (18)

Clinical classification	Number of patients		Hildreth score $\log_{10}\left(\dfrac{\text{after}}{\text{before}} + 10\right)$		Depression rating $\log_{10}\left(\dfrac{\text{before}}{\text{after}} + 10\right)$		Anxiety rating $\log_{10}\left(\dfrac{\text{before}}{\text{after}} + 10\right)$	
	rapid	slow	rapid	slow	rapid	slow	rapid	slow
Neurotic depression	9	15	1.0663 ± 0.0068	1.0784 ± 0.0082	1.1292 ± 0.0330	1.1432 ± 0.0274	1.1044 ± 0.0260	1.1501 ± 0.0280
Endogenous depression	8	15	1.0576 ± 0.0040	1.0837 ± 0.0113	1.0701 ± 0.0127	1.1311 ± 0.0403	1.0758 ± 0.0150	1.0968 ± 0.0157
All patients	17	30	1.0622 ± 0.0039	1.0811 ± 0.0068	1.1014 ± 0.0200	1.1371 ± 0.0240	1.0909 ± 0.0153	1.1234 ± 0.0165
			t = 1.970 p < 0.10		t = 1.015 p > 0.10		t = 1.309 p > 0.10	

Reproduced by kind permission of Prof. *D.A. Price Evans*, Liverpool.

Table III. Incidence of adverse effects in phenelzine therapy (trial of *Evans et al.*, 18)

Acetylator phenotype	Adverse effects			Total
	nil	slight	severe	
Rapid	12	5	0	17
Slow	16	6	9	31
Total	28	11	9	48

Reproduced by kind permission of Prof. *D.A. Price Evans*, Liverpool.

studied the response of 47 depressed patients to a 4-week course of phenelzine, given in a dose of 15 mg t.i.d. The acetylator phenotype was determined by an isoniazid loading method prior to treatment being begun and ratings of depression and anxiety were carried out before and after treatment. The group consisted of 17 fast acetylators and 30 slow. 23 of the patients were classed as having endogenous depression and 24 as having neurotic depression. Full details of the patients and their response to phenelzine are contained in tables I—III. Assessment of the psychiatric state was made by means of the Hamilton anxiety and depression scales and by means of the Hildreth self-rating feeling attitude scale (19—21). Side-effects were recorded only if they were spontaneously reported. No significant differences were found in clinical improvement between the two phenotypes but severe side-effects were reported only by slow acetylators although slight side-effects occurred in both groups. This distribution of side-effects supported the idea that phenelzine was subject to polymorphic acetylation in human populations but this study gave no evidence to suggest that acetylator phenotype was related to the anti-depressant effect of the drug. The findings of the Medical Research Council (MRC) study in 1965 suggested that phenelzine would not benefit endogenously depressed patients (16) who comprised half of the population of this study. *Johnstone and Marsh* (22) in 1973 carried out a 6-week double-blind cross-over trial of phenelzine versus placebo in 72 patients with neurotic depression and related the response of these patients to their acetylator phenotype. Each patient had 1 week on phenelzine 15 mg t.i.d. followed by 2 weeks on phenelzine 30 mg t.i.d. either before or after 3 weeks of placebo. The sample consisted of 39 slow acetylators and 33 fast. The mental state was assessed by means of a modification of the standardised psychiatric interview devised by *Goldberg et al.* (23) (table IV). These two groups did not differ in age or placebo response but they did differ in response to phenelzine. A trend whereby phenelzine was more effective as an anti-depressant in slow acetylators than in fast was shown throughout the study and at times this achieved statistical significance. The trial showed that for fast

Table IV. Modified Goldberg score

Symptom areas	depression anxiety phobias obsessions and compulsions
Manifest abnormalities	depressed anxious
Overall severity =	symptom score + (manifest abnormality score × 2)

Table V. Comparison between response of fast and slow acetylators to placebo and phenelzine (trial of *Johnstone and Marsh,* 22)

Drug	Fast acetylators	Slow acetylators	p^1
Week 3 scores:			
Placebo	5.83 ± 4.43 (n = 23)	8.39 ± 5.79 (n = 23)	NS
Phenelzine	5.80 ± 4.55 (n = 10)	2.18 ± 2.48 (n = 16)	< 0.025
Week 3 to week 6 differences:			
Placebo	0.60 ± 3.53 (n = 10)	1.00 ± 2.96 (n = 16)	NS
Phenelzine	4.39 ± 4.78 (n = 23)	6.69 ± 4.73 (n = 23)	NS

1 By Student's t-test. NS = not significant.

Table VI. Efficacy of drug versus placebo in fast and slow acetylators: week 0 to week 3 differences (trial of *Johnstone and Marsh,* 22)

Acetylator status	Placebo	Phenelzine	p^1
Slow	7.13 ± 4.70 (n = 23)	12.06 ± 5.10 (n = 16)	< 0.0025
Fast	8.13 ± 5.42 (n = 23)	11.30 ± 6.40	NS

1 By Student's t-test. NS = not significant.

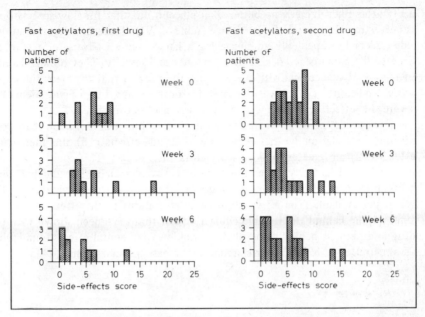

Fig. 1. Side-effects of fast acetylators (trial of *Johnstone and Marsh,* 22).

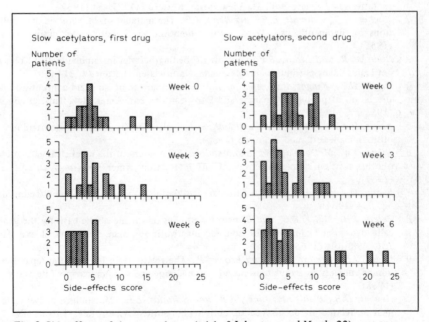

Fig. 2. Side-effects of slow acetylators (trial of *Johnstone and Marsh,* 22).

acetylators phenelzine is no better than placebo but that for slow acetylators it is better to a highly significant degree (table V, VI). These investigators studied side-effects by repeatedly administering a list of known adverse effects of the drug to the patients and noting their presence and severity. They obtained a high incidence of side-effects with placebo and they found that the mean side-effect score while on the drug was the same for both groups, but a few patients had severe side-effects and these were mainly slow acetylators (fig. 1, 2).

The results of these two studies suggest that phenelzine is subject to polymorphic acetylation in that they show that side-effects (18) and therapeutic effects (22) are greater in slow acetylators than in fast. This could be held to imply that this is likely to be because more active phenelzine is available to slow acetylators than to fast for any given dosage of the drug. Direct evidence for this is not yet available. The relevance of acetylator status to the effects of phenelzine may lie behind the variable clinical effects that have been shown with this drug and perhaps behind some of the variable experimental effects found when administration of MAOI is correlated with increase in brain amines (24).

References

1 *Robitzek, E.H.; Selikoff, I.J., and Ornstein, G.G.:* Chemotherapy of human tuberculosis with hydrazine derivatives of isonicotinic acid. A preliminary report of representative cases. Quart. Bull. Sea View Hosp., N.Y. *13* (1): 27–51 (1952).

2 *Hughes, H.B.; Schmidt, L.H., and Biehl, J.P.:* The metabolism of isoniazid, its implications in therapeutic use. Trans. Conf. Chemotherap. Tuberc., Washington *14:* 217 (1955).

3 *Bonicke, R. und Lisboa, B.P.:* Über die Erbbedingtheit der intraindividuellen Konstanz der Isoniazidausscheidung beim Menschen. Naturwissenschaften *44:* 314 (1957).

4 *Harris, H.W.; Knight, R.A., and Selin, M.J.:* Comparison of isoniazid concentrations in the blood of people of Japanese and European descent. Amer. Rev. Tuberc. *78:* 944 (1958).

5 *Evans, D.A.P.; Manley, K.A., and McKusick, V.A.:* Genetic control of isoniazid metabolism in man. Brit. med. J. *ii:* 485 (1960).

6 *Jenne, J.W.; McDonald, F.M., and Mendoza, E.:* A study of the renal clearances metabolic inactivation rates and serum fall off interaction. Amer. Rev. resp. Dis. *84:* 371 (1961).

7 *Evans, D.A.P. and White, T.A.:* Human acetylation polymorphism. J. Lab. clin. Med. *63:* 394 (1964).

8 *Peters, J.H.; Miller, K.S., and Brown, P.:* Studies on the metabolic basis for the genetically determined capacities for isoniazid inactivation in man. J. Pharmacol. exp. Ther. *150:* 298–304 (1965).

9 *Peters, J.H.; Gordon, G.R., and Brown, P.:* The relationship between the capacities of human subjects to acetylate isoniazid sulfanilamide and sulfamethazine. Life Sci. *4:* 99 (1965).

10 *Hughes, H.B.; Biehl, J.P.; Jones, A.P., and Schmidt, L.H.:* Metabolism of isoniazid in man as related to occurrence of peripheral neuritis. Amer. Rev. Tuberc. *70:* 266 (1954).

11 *Devadatta, S.; Gangadharam, P.R.J.; Andrews, R.H.; Fox, W.; Ramakrishnan, C.V.; Selkon, J.B., and Velu, S.:* Peripheral neuritis due to isoniazid. Bull. Wld Hlth Org. *23:* 587 (1960).

12 *Jenne, J.W.:* Partial purification and properties of the isoniazid transacetylase in human liver. Its relationship to the acetylation of *p*-aminosalicylic acid. J. clin. Invest. *44:* 1992 (1965).

13 *Smirnov, G.A. and Kozulitzina, T.I.:* Relation of the toxic action of phthivazid to the nature of its conversion in the body. Vop. Med. Khim. *8:* 401–406 (1962).

14 *Spector, S.; Prockop, D.; Shore, P.A., and Brodie, B.B.:* Effect of iproniazid on brain levels of norpinephrine and serotonin. Science *127:* 704 (1958).

15 *McLean, R.; Nicholson, W.J.; Pare, C.M.B., and Stacey, R.S.:* Effect of monoamine oxidase inhibitors on the concentrations of 5-hydroxytryptamine in the human brain. Lancet *ii:* 205–208 (1965).

16 British Medical Journal: Clinical trial of the treatment of depressive illness. Report to the Medical Research Council by its Clinical Psychiatry Committee. Brit. med. J. *i:* 881 (1965).

17 *Pare, C.M.B., Rees, L., and Sainsbury, M.J.:* Differentiation of two genetically specific types of depression by the response to antidepressants. Lancet *ii:* 1340 (1962).

18 *Evans, D.A.P.; Davidson, K., and Pratt, R.T.C.:* The influence of acetylator phenotype on the effects of treating depression with phenelzine. Clin. Pharmacol. Ther. *6:* 430 (1965).

19 *Hamilton, M.:* The assessment of anxiety states by rating. Brit. J. med. Psychol. *32:* 50–55 (1959).

20 *Hamilton, M.:* A rating scale for depression. J. Neurol. Neurosurg. Psychiat. *23:* 56–62 (1960).

21 *Hildreth, H.M.:* A battery of feeling and attitude scales for clinical use. J. clin. Psychol. *2:* 214–221 (1946).

22 *Johnstone, E.C. and Marsh, W.:* Acetylator status and response to phenelzine in depressed patients. Lancet *i:* 567–570 (1973).

23 *Goldberg, D.P.; Cooper, B.; Eastwood, M.R.; Kedward, H.B., and Shepherd, M.:* A standardised psychiatric interview for use in community surveys. Brit. J. prev. soc. Med. *24:* 18–23 (1970).

24 *Bevan Jones, A.B.; Pare, C.M.B.; Nicholson, W.J.; Price, K., and Stacey, R.S.:* Brain amine concentrations after monoamine oxidase inhibitor administration. Brit. med. J. *i:* 17–19 (1972).

Dr. *Eve C. Johnstone,* Department of Psychological Medicine, University of Glasgow, and Southern General Hospital, *Glasgow, G51 4TF* (Scotland)

Genetics and Psychopharmacology. Mod. Probl. Pharmacopsych., vol. 10, pp. 38–56, ed. *J. Mendlewicz*, Brussels (Karger, Basel 1975)

Low Platelet Monoamine Oxidase and Vulnerability to Schizophrenia

Richard J. Wyatt, Robert Belmaker and Dennis Murphy

Laboratory of Clinical Psychopharmacology, Adult Psychiatry Branch, and Laboratory of Clinical Science, National Institute of Mental Health, Bethesda, Md.

I. Introduction

Previous studies (1) had led us to postulate that an abnormality in indole metabolism might be present in schizophrenia, and led us to our examination of several indole-related enzymes in schizophrenic patients (2–4). Since monoamine oxidase (MAO) is a crucial enzyme in the metabolism of both serotonin and tryptamine, our initial finding (2) that MAO was low in the platelets of schizophrenics started us on an extensive exploration to determine which patients had the deficit, whether the deficit was in some way a secondary process to being schizophrenic, the chemical nature of the deficit and whether the deficit was present elsewhere in the body (5–8). It of course does not follow that because there may be a deficit in MAO that there is an abnormality in indoleamine metabolism. Other substrates may be involved. This paper describes some of our current efforts to examine these problems but primarily focuses on our genetic studies.

MAO Assay in Blood Platelets

Venous blood was collected in Becton-Dickinson Co. Vacutainer tubes containing acid-citrate-dextrose (ACD), NIH formula A, and platelets separated and stored according to previously described methods (4). MAO activity was determined using tryptamine-2-^{14}C HCl (8×10^{-5} m, 8.9 mCi/mM) as substrate and is expressed as nanomoles of tryptamine converted per milligram of platelet protein (2). The product is indoleacetaldehyde, whose formation is linear with time and enzyme concentration. Tyramine and benzylamine were also used as substrates for a limited number of subjects.

Reliability of Assay

Because genetic studies require considerable assay reliability we have endeavored to determine what variability to expect with our method. It is clear after using and improving upon the assay during the last 4 years that the variation between separate runs can be moderately high and that each run must contain its own controls. Our means for normal controls over that period of time have run from 6.4 to 5.2, with lower values occurring during the last year. On the same run, however, the average sample variation $-\overline{X}$ of $[(a - b)/(a + b)] \times 100\%$ for the same individual having blood drawn twice during a day is $\pm 9\%$ while that for the same individual drawn 1 week apart is $\pm 17\%$ (6).

Subjects

The normal bloods were drawn from hospital personnel and normal volunteers at both the Clinical Center in Bethesda, Maryland and the William A. White (WAW) Building at St. Elizabeths Hospital in Washington, D.C. The bloods from the acute schizophrenics largely came from a research ward at the Clinical Center while those from the chronic schizophrenic patients came from special research wards at the WAW Building.

Age and Sex

Although *Robinson et al.* (9) reported that females had 10% higher platelet MAO activity than males, in our samples males and females between the age range of 18–50 years are not statistically different. Females under 20 and over 50 years may have higher platelet MAO activity than males.

Drugs

Although early experiments (10) with chlorpromazine in intact systems indicated that chlorpromazine had some effects on amine degradation, this seemed to be due to poor amine accessibility to the enzyme because of alteration in the cell membrane (11). Tricyclic drugs like imipramine, and phenothiazines like chlorpromazine have effects on MAO activity in homogenized systems only in relatively high concentrations. To test *in vivo* activity in the presence of chlorpromazine 17 chronic schizophrenics on our research wards were taken off all drugs for at least 1 month and their platelets sampled for MAO activity. The same patients were placed on chlorpromazine (400 mg/24 h) for

3 weeks and again their platelets were sampled. The mean ± SEM for the drug-free patients was 2.8 ± 0.60, while that for the patients on chlorpromazine was 2.8 ± 0.43 (2). Nevertheless, for reasons that are not clear (perhaps multiple batches), the average sample variation across individuals from the first to the second assay was high (45 %). Six depressed patients were studied prior to and during treatment (18–76 days) with thioridazine (100–600 mg/24 h). The means were 5.24 ± 0.69 and 5.47 ± 0.82, respectively (6).

Hormones

One study using only two points found no alteration in platelet MAO activity during the human menstrual cycle (12). In a study which we have just completed which utilized samples collected 3 times a week, there were small (23 %) peak-to-trough variations in activity in the majority of women (13). The peak MAO activity occurred during the preovulatory interval and the nadir occurred 5–11 days later. A small number of patients taking prednisone have been seen and have normal MAO activities (6).

Chronic Schizophrenics

To date we have studied platelet MAO activity in 68 chronic schizophrenic patients (fig. 1). Their mean MAO activity was 2.86 ± 0.25, while the values for 181 normals (ages 18–40 years) were 5.24 ± 0.20. This difference, using a 2-tailed t-test, is significant at $p < 0.001$. The mean for the 53 male chronic schizophrenics was 2.91 ± 0.30, while that for 79 normal males was 5.12 ± 0.32 ($p < 0.001$). The mean for the 15 female chronic schizophrenics was 2.72 ± 0.49, while that for 102 normals was 5.34 ± 0.26 ($p < 0.001$). To date we have not been able to find systematic differences related to length of illness or hospitalization. By our definition, the chronic schizophrenic patients have a minimum hospitalization period of at least 1 year and have been ill for at least 2 years. Furthermore, there are no clear differences in platelet MAO activity between schizophrenic subtypes. Further investigations to attempt to determine psychosocial relationship among the normal and low platelet MAO patients are under way.

Acute versus Chronic Schizophrenics

To determine whether acute schizophrenics have a reduction in platelet MAO as did the chronic schizophrenics, platelet MAO of 27 acute schizophrenics (fig. 1) free from all drugs for at least 2 weeks were studied. These patients were

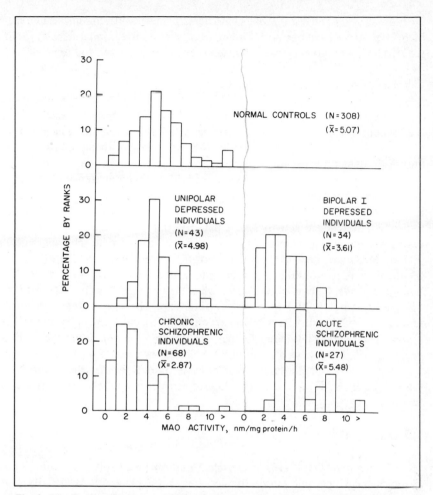

Fig. 1. Distribution frequency of platelet monoamine oxidase (MAO) activity in normal, unipolar depressed, bipolar I depressed, chronic schizophrenic and acute schizophrenic patients. Normal populations throughout the paper when compared to other groups are matched for age. The 308 normal subjects here are all those above 16 years that we have studied.

housed on a special National Institute of Mental Health (NIMH) research ward in Bethesda, supervised by Dr. *William Carpenter* (14). The acute schizophrenics (ages 16–30 years) had a mean platelet MAO activity of 5.48 ± 0.44 which was no different from that for 181 age-matched normals (5.24 ± 0.70). The 11 male acute patients had a mean of 4.56 ± 0.45 which was no different from that for

79 normal males (5.12 ± 0.30). The 16 female acute schizophrenics had a mean of 6.11 ± 0.64 which was no different from that of 102 normal females (5.34 ± 0.27). There were no subgrouping differences in the acute schizophrenics.

Specificity with Regard to Other Illness

A usual strategy in psychiatric research once a given effect is established in one patient group is to look at other diagnostic groups for the same alteration. Since the various diagnostic classifications are thought to represent different entities, a defect in one should not be seen in the other. The depressive illnesses are the group we most diligently contrasted with the schizophrenias (15).

43 unipolar depressed patients (fig. 1) were found to have platelet MAO activity that was no different from our controls while 34 bipolar I depressed patients[1] had reduced activity (3.6 ± 0.32 p < 0.001. The bipolar patients had a negative skew which was not as large as that of the chronic schizophrenics. If 2 U of MAO are used as a point of cutoff, a point under which 40 % ($\chi^2 = 33.46$, df = 1; p > 0.001) of the chronic schizophrenics fit, we find 7 of 34 bipolar patients. This is about 20 %, which is not significantly different ($\chi^2 = 2.69$, df = 1; p > 0.001) than that for controls. There was no significant difference ($\chi^2 = 2.47$, df = 1; p > 0.1) between the chronic schizophrenics and the bipolar I patients. Thus, even though the bipolar I patients using the arbitrary cutoff of 2 U MAO have a mean MAO which is low, it is not yet clear whether they represent a separate group. It is possible, therefore, that the factors which lower platelet MAO in the chronic schizophrenic and bipolar patients are different.

Confirmation

Meltzer and Stahl (16), studying 15 normal controls, 10 acute schizophrenics and 12 chronic schizophrenics, found low platelet MAO activity, using tryptamine and octopamine as substrates in the chronic schizophrenics only. However, using metaidobenzylamine and tyramine, both the acute and chronic patients were found to have low platelet MAO activity. Our own studies using tyramine as a substrate in 10 chronic schizophrenic patients produced mean activities in pmoles per milligram protein per hour of 17.8 ± 1.95. The activities for 16 acute schizophrenics were 36.2 ± 3.86 while that for 19 normal controls was 37.5 ± 4.95. The differences between the chronic schizophrenics and controls is highly significant (p < 0.01).

---

1   Bipolar depressed patients were differentiated from unipolar depressed patients on the basis of the occurrence of mania severe enough to require hospitalization or specific treatment in the bipolar patients.

Table I. Platelet monoamine oxidase (MAO) activity in monozygotic twins discordant for schizophrenia

Twin pair	Age	Sex	Diagnosis, τ		Platelet MAO activity, nM/mg protein/h	
			index	non-schizophrenic	index	non-schizophrenic
1	33	F	CUS	none	5.59[1]	7.98
2	30	M	CUS	none	3.98[1]	2.79
5	37	M	CPS	none	4.02[1]	9.49
7	34	F	AUS in remission	none	5.61[1]	5.12
8	30	M	CPS	none	0.64	1.64
10	42	F	CPS	none	5.47	8.49
14	25	F	CUS in partial remission	none	1.63	1.58
17	37	F	CPS	none	0.31[1]	1.77
18	51	F	APS in remission	none	5.33	4.14
22	35	F	CPS in remission	none	5.57[1]	7.19
23	31	M	CUS	borderline	1.56	0.72
21	44	F	AUS in remission	none	7.64[1]	4.79
26	55	M	APS in remission	none	4.13	4.54

τ diagnosis: CUS = chronic undifferentiated schizophrenia; CPS = chronic paranoid schizophrenia; AUS = acute undifferentiated schizophrenia; APS = acute paranoid schizophrenia.
1 Patients receiving phenothiazine drugs.

Twins Discordant for Schizophrenia

To exclude the possibility that the low platelet MAO activity seen in the chronic schizophrenics was caused by nongenetic factors as opposed to genetic ones, we studied monozygotic twins discordant for schizophrenia (5). If the low platelet MAO activity is due to some aspect of being schizophrenic, low platelet MAO should only be present in the schizophrenic twin. 13 schizophrenic index twins, all of whom had been hospitalized at least once for schizophrenia, and had been extensively studied by Dr. *William Pollin* and his associates, were examined along with their nonschizophrenic co-twins (table I). At the time of the study, one patient resided within a hospital while 5 were in remission. Four of the patients had had acute forms of schizophrenia and 6 patients were not receiving any antipsychotic medication. The nonschizophrenic co-twins had never been hospitalized for a behavioral disorder and were functioning well within their families and communities, except for one individual with borderline psychosocial adjustment.

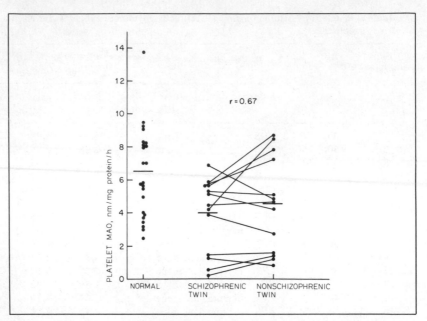

Fig. 2. MAO activity in 23 normal and 13 pairs of monozygotic twins discordant for schizophrenia. Correlation is between discordant twins (p < 0.01).

Only 2 twin pairs were living in the same household and 9 of the co-twins were living in different cities. It was, therefore, necessary to obtain and prepare the blood samples at various facilities throughout the country. Because of this, normal control samples were obtained at the same time as those from the twins. They were coded and shipped to the laboratory. All samples were batched together before assay. (In all studies samples are run in a manner so that their origins are unknown to all investigators until the final calculations are made.)

The MAO activity of the 23 normal controls (fig. 2) was the same as that obtained for previous controls (6.4 ± 0.562 SEM). The schizophrenic twins (3.9 ± 0.638 SEM, p < 0.005) and nonschizophrenic twins (4.7 ± 0.804 SEM, p < 0.05) were significantly lower than the normals, but there was no difference between the twin groups (table I). There was a significant Pearson correlation (r = 0.67, p < 0.01) between the MAO activities in the schizophrenic and non-schizophrenic twins.

Examination of figure 2 reveals that there are 4 pairs of twins whose MAO activities are below 2 U. The indexes of all 4 of these twin pairs are chronic schizophrenics while the more acute patients have MAO activities closer to normal. The severity of impairment (based upon number and duration of hospitalizations) was rated on a 5-point scale for the schizophrenic twins by an investigator with no knowledge of the platelet assay. A forced rank order was then made between the numerical ratings, with the highest number given to the most-ill patient. Using this order, and comparing it to the MAO activities, a Spearman rank order correlation of -0.54 ($p < 0.05$) was found.

Platelet MAO activity was also examined in 9 monozygotic and 10 dizygotic normal twins (6). The intraclass correlation coefficient was 0.88 for the monozygotic and 0.45 for the dizygotic twins. The correlations were significantly different from one another (Mann Whitney U $p < 0.001$). Same-sex siblings matched for age and sex were about the same as the dizygotic twins while unrelated pairs were not significantly correlated with each other (6). These results are similar to those reported by *Nies et al.* (17) for normal monozygotic and dizygotic twins using benzylamine instead of tryptamine as a substrate.

Taken together this data indicates that platelet MAO activity is in a large part determined by genetic factors and that the low platelet MAO activity seen in the chronic schizophrenics is not secondary to being ill, but is genetically related to the liability to be schizophrenic.

Family Studies

In order to study further the relationship of low platelet MAO to schizophrenia the blood of first degree relatives of index schizophrenics (N = 10) was collected. Using schizophrenic indexes (N = 7) with low MAO (mean 1.99) the mean MAO activity for the first-degree relatives (N = 27) was 3.22. The mean activity for first-degree relatives (N = 15) of patients with high MAO activity (N = 3, mean = 5.55) was 5.19. The Pearson correlation between indexes (N = 12 including 2 psychologically normal families) and first-degree relatives (N = 44) was 0.73.

Since an individual can expect to have no more than half his inheritance the same as any other relative, a maximum correlation of 0.5 was expected. Therefore, a 0.73 correlation between indexes and the mean value for their first-degree relatives needs an explanation. The first explanation is that the high correlation represents a random statistical error. Another possible explanation is that we have inadvertently introduced a systematic error in preparing our platelets. This could happen if families came in as a group (they did) and we varied the platelet preparation from family to family. A third possibility would occur if there were strong intrafamily environmental factors altering platelet MAO. A fourth possibility is that there is assortive mating of the parents which is supported by a 0.57 correlation between mates in the 8 couples we have data on. The latter finding, however, could be explained by any of the first 3 reasons. This experiment will have to be repeated to determine which of these factors is producing this effect.

Physical-Chemical Studies

To date we have found no physical differences between the low and normal platelet MAO, The K_ms from 6 schizophrenic patients (all below 3.1 U) and from 8 normals were nearly identical (4.1 × 10^{-5} and 4.3 × 10^{-5} M). The heat inactivation curves for both groups showed reductions in activity at 50 °C which were not different for the 2 groups. The platelet MAO is not easily solubilized which has, to date, prevented reliable electrophoretic studies. Dialysis of platelet sonicates from 10 schizophrenic patients and 7 controls did not reveal any postdialysis differences in activity between schizophrenic patients and controls (2).

II. Mode of Inheritance

Possible Sex Effect and X-Linkage

Because our research wards have preselected male patients, the vast majority of the chronic schizophrenic patients in our studies are male. Thus, the low MAO activity in our sampling has largely been confined to male patients. Of the 15 female patients in this sample, however, 7 are below an arbitrary 2 U under which 40 % of the male chronic schizophrenic patients also fit. Similarly there is no difference in the low distribution between males (14/104) and females (11/126) of our normal group (18–30 years) or between male (0/11) and female (0/16) acute schizophrenics.

Another approach to this problem has been to study a large family (family C) with low platelet MAO activity and multiple psychoses versus relation to the Xg^a antigen (18). The Xg^a antigen is a red cell antigen whose genetic locus is on the X chromosome which in certain families is genetically linked to the presence or absence of manic-depressive illness (19). In family C (table II), which included a mother and 9 living children, the probability of X-linked inheritance of the psychosis is 0.83 (binomial test). The father could not be examined but the finding that both male and female offspring have low MAO activity (with one exception) suggests that if low MAO is X-linked both the mother and father had one X-linked recessive gene. If both parents have one X-linked recessive gene producing low MAO, one-half the females should be low. Instead 3 of 4 are low. One-half the males should also be low, receiving one of the 2 X chromosomes from the mother. All 4 male children, however, are low. The probability of 7 (3 female and 4 males) of 8 things happening when only 4 (2 female and 2 male) of 8 are expected is 0.03. Thus, it seems unlikely that platelet MAO activity is controlled by a gene on the X chromosome even though in this family psychosis may be linked to it.

Table II. Family C with multiple psychotic individuals. Likelihood of an X-chromosome linkage of psychosis and demonstrating unlikelihood of X-chromosome linkage of platelet MAO activity

Relationship	Sex	Age, years	Status	Xg[a]	Platelet MAO activity, nM/mg/protein/h
Father	M	deceased	alcoholic		
Mother	F	65	psychotic depression	+ –	3.19
Son	M	44	bipolar manic-depressive	–	2.06
Daughter	F	deceased	*postpartum* suicide		
Daughter	F	38	no psychosis	++	
Daughter	F	36	no psychosis	+ –	2.75
Son	M	35	psychotic depression	–	1.54
Daughter	F	32	no psychosis	++	2.70
Son	M	30	acute schizophrenia	+	2.36
Daughter	F	30	no psychosis	++	5.78
Son	M	27	schizo-affective	–	2.27
Daughter	F	27	schizo-affective	+ –	1.92

binomial test probability of X-linking inheritance of psychosis is 0.83

binomial test probability of there being X-linkage of MAO is 0.03

The mode of transmission for platelet MAO activity is not evident but there are several tools available to examine it.

Dominant Transmission

In a dominant or nearly dominant single gene inheritance, one of the parents of an index should have almost the exact deficit seen in the index. We do not see this in family F (fig. 3). The index male has platelet MAO activity of 1.51 while his mother and father (also schizophrenic) have MAO activity of 3.72 and 3.96, respectively. Of course, many more families need to be studied before definite conclusions excluding a dominant transmission model can be made. Family G may show a similar inconsistency. An index father has MAO activity of 1.03 and a mother has 3.36. In the 5 offspring we would expect at least 2 of the children to have an MAO value as low as the father, while the closest is 1.41.

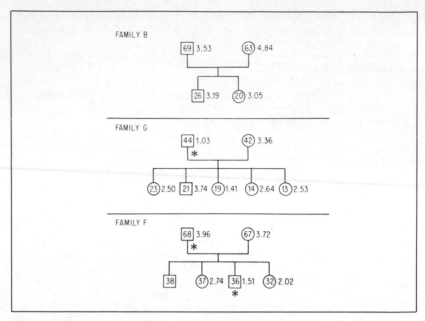

Fig. 3. Diagram of 3 families and values of platelet MAO activity. Numbers inside circles (female) or boxes (male) are ages. Star = schizophrenic.

Recessive Transmission

If a genetic trait is produced by a single recessive gene then it would be expected to appear much more often in the sibs (who are exposed to the same genetic pool as the indexes) than in parents or children (exposed to one-half the genetic pool the sibs and index are exposed to). When we look at the 7 families with index MAO values under 4 U (including one normal family), the mean for the 7 indexes is 2.14, that for the 15 sibs is 3.24 and that for the 15 parents and children is 3.13. The sibs who should be closer to the indexes if a recessive model was operative are actually slightly further away than the parents and children.

Two or More Genes

If platelet MAO activity is neither controlled by a dominant or recessive gene, then two or more genes control it. (The fragmentary evidence above is not intended as a proof but is simply suggestive of some ways family data may be of use.) In a 2-gene model one of these genes might control the MAO rate of production while another might control its destruction rate or perhaps its critical binding to a membrane.

The multiple-gene theory would be supported if a clear dominant or recessive pattern could be shown in one family but not others. For example, if the gene controlling the formation of low MAO was dominant while degradation was normal, this might show up in one family. Such a pattern might be the case in family B (fig. 3) in which the index MAO activity is 3.19, his sister 3.05, his father 3.53 and his mother 4.84. The father and children might have a dominant gene causing slow MAO synthesis, but normal degradation. Another family could have rapid degradation while, still others, slow synthesis and rapid degradation.

Another approach to this problem is to use median split analysis as described by *Rosenthal* (20). The test would involve 2 substantial groups of persons, all of whom had children. One group would consist of schizophrenics serving as indexes, the second of matched controls. If low monoamine oxidase is produced by more than one gene, then not only should the offspring of schizophrenics as a group have lower MAO activity but if the sibs are split at their medians, both those schizophrenic offspring above and below the median should be lower than the control offspring. On the other hand, a single gene that was dominant or nearly dominant (present in only one-half the children of schizophrenics) would produce low MAO activity in only one-half the children of schizophrenics and the other half should be identical to the control children.

Relationship of Platelet MAO to Brain MAO

There is some conflict over how many MAO are present in the brain. Although the original studies (21) indicated that there might be as many as 4 isoenzymes of MAO within the brain, recently *Houslay and Tipton* (22) suggested that the multiple enzymes found using polyacrylamide gel electrophoresis might be produced in a preparatory step. The authors state that these multiple MAO forms may represent a single protein with varying amounts of phospholipid attached; the amount of phospholipid may in turn determine the enzyme mobility during electrophoresis.

Another approach to this problem has come from the finding that selective inhibition of MAO can be used to identify multiple forms of MAO. Clorgyline was the first MAO inhibitor employed in this manner (23). It was found that tissue homogenates pretreated with increasing concentrations of clorgyline produced stepwise inhibition to the substrate tyramine, suggesting the presence of an enzyme sensitive to the inhibitor and one relatively resistent to it. Considerably more work has been done to identify these enzymes and for convenience they are called type A and type B (24).

The preferred substrates for the type A MAO are norepinephrine, serotonin and normetanephrine, while for type B they are benzylamine and β-phenylethylamine. Dopamine, tyramine and tryptamine are common substrates. Clorgyline, Lilly 51641 and harmaline are specific inhibitors of type A, while deprenyl inhibits type B. Most of the other MAO inhibitors used in clinical medicine, however, are nonspecific. Platelet MAO, forming a single band on electrophoresis, appears to be one enzyme and is more like the type B enzyme than type A, but a full comparison has not yet been made.

MAO in the Brain and Liver of Schizophrenic Patients

Birkhäuser (25), studying the putamen and globus pallidus of 8 schizophrenics and 6 normals, found a 15-percent difference in O_2 production. In 1955, *Takahashi* (26) found a 40-percent increase in biopsied liver tissue in 25 schizophrenic patients compared to 14 nonschizophrenic patients. *Utena et al.* (27), comparing 5 chronic schizophrenics and 15 patients without mental illness, found no difference in brain MAO activity in any of 24 regions studied; however, when the areas were organized into functional units including hypothalamus, tegmentum, and striatum the schizophrenics had lower MAO activity in these regions. Finally, 3 recent studies (28—30) have failed to find differences in brain MAO activity using methods very similar to those used for our platelet assay.

In order to examine further the apparent contradiction described above, we collected 15 regions of autopsied brain from 9 chronic schizophrenics and 9 persons without history of psychiatric illness (7). Using tryptamine as a substrate there was no difference in mean MAO activity in any region examined. The brains were subsequently examined using serotonin and clorgyline to test for MAO A and B, phenylethylamine and deprenyl for MAO B. Again, there were no differences in the mean MAO activity between the schizophrenics and controls (8).

Function

To determine (31) whether or not the low platelet MAO activity might have a functional significance, platelet-rich plasma was obtained from 20 normal controls (age 29.6 ± 1.1 years) and 16 chronic schizophrenic patients (age 27 ± 1.4 years). Since plasma serotonin is almost entirely contained in the platelet the values are expressed in platelet units (ng/10^8 platelets). The platelet counts for the normals and schizophrenics were the same. When the patients had been off phenothiazines (N = 12) for 30 days or longer the serotonin concentration was higher ($p < 0.01$) in the schizophrenics (127 ± 12) than in the normals (80 ± 4), while when the patients were taking phenothiazines ($N = 12$) their platelet serotonin concentration was normal (90 ± 9). The reason for the discrepancy between patients taking and not taking phenothiazines may be due to the ability of the latter to block serotonin uptake into platelets.

MAO and Another Deficit?

If recent estimates of concordance for chronic schizophrenia in monozygotic twins are correct at about 40 %, then 60 % of schizophrenic genocopies do not become schizophrenic phenocopies. Assuming an incidence of schizophrenia of 1 % in the population, 2.5 % of the population are genetically at as much risk as the 1 % that become schizophrenic. If one half of the 1 % who are schizophrenic are chronic schizophrenics and one-half of these have a deficit in MAO, somewhat less than 1 % of the general population would be susceptible to 'low MAO chronic schizophrenia'. Assuming that our 'control' 10 % with low MAO activity is representative of the general population, then the schizophrenic genotype is at least one-tenth the expected value. This could indicate that a second deficit is needed to produce schizophrenia.

If the following simplifying assumptions are made: (1) that a model with two genes is involved; (2) that our control population is representative of the real population; (3) that 10 % of the control population has low MAO activity and therefore has the genetic defect; (4) that 1 % of the population is schizophrenic; (5) that they are all chronic schizophrenics, and (6) that 40 % of the chronic schizophrenic population has low MAO activity and that this is a genetic defect, then the incidence of the second genetic defect (I_2) in the general population must be in the order of 4 % ($I_2 = 40 \times 1/10$ %). When other numbers are used, slightly different incidences of the second defect are found. For example, if 20 % of the normal population and 60 % of the schizophrenic population are used then the second deficit should be present in 3 % of the general population. If it is thought that only one-half of the 1 % of schizophrenics are chronic then the second defect is present in only 2 % of the normal population. Whatever the exact incidence of the second deficit, it would have to be small.

With regard to schizophrenia, there is currently little agreement whether it is due to recessive, dominant, or multiple genes; however, a great number of psychologically normal people have had their MAO activity reduced by exogenous inhibitors of the enzyme and it seems that more than low enzyme activity is required to produce schizophrenia. This is because the rate of psychosis in persons taking MAO inhibitors for angina and hypertension is low (32). The incidence of psychosis for patients taking ipronizid may be as high as 10–20 %, but this drug may have other biological effects besides its MAO-inhibiting properties. The reasons for this low rate with other MAO inhibitors may be that the patients have not taken the drug long enough, or the low activity has not occurred at the appropriate time in their life or that a second factor is needed.

Schizophrenia Spectrum Disorder

Kety et al. (33) have introduced the concept of the schizophrenia spectrum disorders — a higher than usual prevalence of schizophrenia-related illnesses in family members of schizophrenics. They used adoption to separate genetic and environmental factors in the transmission of schizophrenia among family members. They found a high prevalence of schizophrenia-related illnesses among biological relatives of adopted schizophrenics but not among their adoptive relatives. In their study of 16 chronic schizophrenics with 82 relatives, 7 of the relatives were chronic schizophrenics, borderline or inadequate personalities. Similarly, their study of 10 borderline schizophrenics with 38 relatives revealed 6 relatives which fit into one of these diagnostic categories. None of the relatives were acute schizophrenics and none of the 30 relatives of the 7 acute schizophrenics were chronic schizophrenics, acute schizophrenics, borderline or inadequate personalities.

The apparent dissociation between chronic and acute schizophrenics in the adoptive studies is also present in our studies of platelet MAO activity in which no difference was found between the acute schizophrenics and our normal controls. In a study of 15,909 veteran twin pairs (34), data was obtained on 234 where an assignment of bipolar or schizophrenic illness could be made in at least one member of the pair. While a concordance rate of 38.5 and 23.5 was obtained for the monozygotic bipolar and schizophrenic twins, respectively, and 0 and 5.3 for the dizygotic twins, there was no twin pair in which one twin was schizophrenic while the other was bipolar. In fact, there appears to be no case in the literature of one twin being schizophrenic while his co-twin is bipolar (35). Thus, our finding that bipolar I patients have low MAO activity but which may not, however, be as low as our chronic schizophrenics is consistent with a schizophrenic spectrum disorder excluding the bipolar illness.

The concept of a schizophrenia spectrum of personality disorders suggested that low platelet MAO might be found in individuals with schizophrenia-related personality patterns. Co-twins of schizophrenics have both low platelet MAO and a high frequency of emotional disorders, even in pairs discordant for schizophrenia itself. The Danish adoption studies found a high prevalence of schizophrenia spectrum disorders, about 15 %, in controls. We therefore decided to study the relationship between platelet MAO and personality patterns among individuals without a history of psychiatric treatment (36). 95 normal volunteers were studied, 30 males and 65 females. The instruments chosen were the Minnesota multiphasic personality inventory (MMPI) and the Zuckerman test, because several scales of these tests have been shown in twin studies to measure heritable components of personality.

Among males, multiple correlation of scales D, Pe and Sc (scales likely to be elevated with chronic schizophrenia) was significantly associated with low platelet MAO. The Zuckerman Z scale, measuring sensation-seeking or impulsive feelings, was also significantly associated with low platelet MAO ($r = -0.45$, $p < 0.05$). Eight of the other 11 MMPI scales also correlated negatively with platelet MAO, although these differences were not statistically significant. Among females, only the paranoia scale correlated negatively with platelet MAO while hypochondriasis and psychasthenia correlated positively ($p < 0.05$). Only 7 % of females had platelet MAO activities below 2.75 nm/mg/h, however, whereas 23 % of the males did. These studies in normals suggest the possibility that platelet MAO activity may correlate with some given personality functions, some of which (especially in males) may be relevant to factors in schizophrenia.

III. Discussion

The data relating low MAO activity to some patients with schizophrenia is especially exciting because it is consistent with the two major biochemical theories of schizophrenia, i.e., that there is a functional excess of dopamine or that there is an increased methylation of one of the biogenic amines which, in turn, is a natural hallucinogen. To attempt to tie in one or the other of these theories to the existing data, however, is premature.

Low platelet MAO activity in chronic schizophrenics has been found in 2 laboratories, and adequate time to allow us and other investigators to demonstrate a possible artifactual origin has not elapsed. Some statements about it do seem appropriate. Low platelet MAO as seen in chronic schizophrenia is not universally seen in other patients with psychiatric disorders and is not strictly a function of being hospitalized. Platelet MAO activity is under considerable genetic control but the degree of environmental control is not known. Natural experiments involving measuring its activity in platelets of normal related children (or twins) brought up in the same home *versus* similar related children brought up separately, as well as data about unrelated children brought up in the same home *versus* different homes might give us some handle on the effect of environment.

Assuming the deficit we are observing is real, further efforts are needed to characterize it from the point of view of its physical-chemical properties, function (or lack of it), mode of transmission, how it manifests itself in sickness and health and whether the deficit is present in other organs. As this work progresses it should become possible to determine whether or not other concomitant deficits are needed to produce schizophrenia or whether low platelet MAO schizophrenia is a spectrum of disorders with the widest flanks including persons who are entirely normal. It is clear, however, that whatever future studies reveal in these areas, that there are a large number of chronic schizophrenics with normal platelet MAO for which other causes of illness must be sought. Finally, in the unlikely event that all these 'ifs' take on a certain degree of probability, a prevention or treatment can be sought.

Summary

Low platelet MAO activity has been found in some chronic schizophrenics. This deficit appears at least in part to be genetically determined. The possible genetic transmission of this abnormality has been discussed.

References

1 *Wyatt, R.J.; Termini, B., and Davis, J.:* Biochemistry of schizophrenia 1970. II. Sleep and schizophrenia (the serotonin hypothesis). Schizo. Bull. *4:* 45–66 (1971).

2 *Murphy, D.L. and Wyatt, R.J.:* Reduced MAO activity in blood platelets from schizophrenic patients. Nature, Lond. *238:* 225–226 (1972).

3 *Dunner, D.L.; Cohn, C.K.; Winshilboom, R.M., and Wyatt, R.J.:* The activity of dopamine-beta hydroxylase and methionine activating enzyme in blood of schizophrenic patients. Biol. Psychiat. *6:* 215–220 (1973).

4 *Wyatt, R.J.; Saavedra, J.M., and Axelrod, J.:* A dimethyltryptamine (DMT) forming enzyme in human blood. Amer. J. Psychiat. *130:* 754–760 (1973).

5 *Wyatt, R.J.; Murphy, D.L.; Belmaker, R.; Cohen, S.; Donnelly, C.H., and Pollin, W.:* Reduced monoamine oxidase in platelets. A possible genetic marker for vulnerability to schizophrenia. Science *179:* 916–918 (1973).

6 *Murphy, D.L.; Belmaker, R., and Wyatt, R.J.:* Monoamine oxidase in schizophrenia. J. Psychiat. Res. (in press).

7 *Schwartz, M.; Aikens, A.M., and Wyatt, R.J.:* Monoamine oxidase in brains from schizophrenic and mentally normal individuals. Psychopharmacologia *38:* 319–328 (1974).

8 *Schwartz, M.A.; Wyatt, R.J.; Yang, H.Y.T., and Neff, N.:* Multiple forms of monoamine oxidase in brain. A comparison of enzymatic activity in mentally normal and chronic schizophrenic individuals. Arch. gen. Psychiat. *31:* 557–560 (1974).

9 *Robinson, D.S.; Davis, J.M.; Nies, A.; Ravaris, C.L., and Sylwester, D.:* Relation of sex and aging to monoamine oxidase activity of human brain, plasma, and platelets. Arch. gen. Psychiat. *24:* 536 (1971).

10 *Pletscher, A. und Gey, K.F.:* Wirkung von Chlorpromazin auf pharmakologische Veränderungen des 5-Hydroxy-Tryptamin- und Noradrenalin-Gehaltes im Gehirn. Med. exp. *2:* 259–265 (1960).

11 *Gey, K.F. and Pletscher, A.:* Interference of chlorpromazine with the metabolism of aromatic amino-acids in rat brain. Nature, Lond. *194:* 387 (1962).

12 *Gilmore, N.J.; Robinson, D.S.; Nies, A.; Sylwester, D., and Ravaris, C.J.:* Blood mono-

amine oxidase levels in pregnancy and during the menstrual cycle. J. psychosom. Res. *15:* 215–219 (1971).

13 *Belmaker, R.; Murphy, D.L.; Wyatt, R.J., and Loriaux, D.L.:* Human platelet mono-amine oxidase changes during the menstrual cycle. Arch. gen. Psychiat. *31:* 553–556 (1974).

14 *Carpenter, W.; Murphy, D., and Wyatt, R.J.:* Platelet monoamine oxidase and acute schizophrenia. Amer. J. Psychiat. (in press).

15 *Murphy, D.L. and Weiss, R.:* Reduced monoamine oxidase activity in blood platelets from bipolar depressed patients. Amer. J. Psychiat. *128:* 35–41 (1972).

16 *Meltzer, H.Y. and Stahl, S.M.:* Platelet monoamine oxidase activity and substrate preferences in schizophrenic patients. Res. Common Chem. Pathol. Pharmacol. *7:* 419–431 (1974).

17 *Nies, A.; Robinson, D.S.; Lamborn, K.R., and Lampert, R.P.:* Genetic control of platelet and plasma monoamine oxidase activity. Arch. gen. Psychiat. *28:* 834–838 (1973).

18 *Belmaker, R. and Wyatt, R.J.:* Possible X-linkage in a family with varied psychoses (submitted for publication).

19 *Mendlewicz, J.; Fleiss, J.L., and Fieve, R.R.:* Evidence for X-linkage in transmission of manic-depressive illness. J. amer. med. Ass. *222:* 1624–1627 (1972).

20 *Rosenthal, D.:* Prospects for research in schizophrenia. IV. Genetic and environmental factors. Hereditary nature of schizophrenia. Neurosci. Res. Program Bull. *10:* 397–403 (1972).

21 *Sandler, M. and Youdim, M.B.H.:* Multiple forms of monoamine oxidase. Functional significance. Pharmacol. Rev. *24:* 331–348 (1972).

22 *Houslay, M.D. and Tipton, K.F.:* The nature of the electrophoretically separable multiple forms of rat liver monoamine oxidase. Biochem. J. *135:* 173–186 (1973).

23 *Johnston, J.P.:* Some observations upon a new inhibitor of monoamine oxidase in brain tissue. Biochem. Pharmacol. *17:* 1285–1297 (1968).

24 *Yang, H.Y.T. and Neff, N.H.:* Beta-phenylethylamine. A specific substrate for type B monoamine oxidase of brain. J. Pharmacol. exp. Ther. *187:* 365–371 (1973).

25 *Birkhäuser, V.H.:* Cholinesterase und mono-aminoxydase im zentralen nervensystem. Schweiz. med. Wschr. *22:* 750–752 (1941).

26 *Takahashi, Y.:* Amine oxidase activity of liver tissues obtained by needle biopsy together with other liver function tests on schizophrenic patients. A preliminary report. Folia psychiat. neurol. jap. *10:* 263 (1955).

27 *Utena, H.; Kanamura, H.; Suda, S.; Nakamura, R.; Machiyama, Y., and Takahashi, R.:* Studies on the regional distribution of the monoamine oxidase activity in the brains of schizophrenic patients. Proc. Japan Acad. *44:* 1078–1083 (1968).

28 *Vogel, W.H.; Orfei, V., and Century, B.:* Activities of enzymes involved in the formation and destruction of biogenic amines in various areas of human brain. J. Pharmacol. exp. Ther. *165:* 195–203 (1969).

29 *Domino, E.F.; Krause, R.R., and Bowers, J.:* Various enzymes involved with putative transmitters. Arch. gen. Psychiat. *29:* 195–201 (1973).

30 *Wise, C.D.; Baden, M.M., and Stein, L.: Post mortem* measurements of enzymes in human brain. Evidence of a central noradrenergic deficit in schizophrenia. J. Psychiat. Res. (in press).

31 *Garelis, E.; Gillin, J.C.; Wyatt, R.J., and Neff, N.:* Elevated blood serotonin concentrations in chronic, unmedicated schizophrenics. A preliminary study (in press).

32 *Price, J. and Hopkinson, G.:* Mono-amine oxidase inhibitors and schizophrenia. Psychiat. clin. *1:* 65–84 (1968).

33 *Kety, S.S.; Rosenthal, D.; Wender, P.H., and Schulsinger, F.:* The types and prevalence of mental illness in the biological and adoptive families of adopted schizophrenics; in *Rosenthal and Kety* The transmission of schizophrenia, pp. 345–391 (Pergamon Press, New York 1968).

34 *Cohen, S.M.; Allen, M.G.; Pollin, W., and Hrubec, Z.:* Relationship of schizo-affective psychosis to manic depressive psychosis and schizophrenia. Arch. gen. Psychiat. *26:* 539–545 (1972).

35 *Rosenthal, D.:* Genetic theory and abnormal behavior (McGraw-Hill, New York 1970).

36 *Belmaker, R.H.; Buchsbaum, M.; Murphy, D.L.; Wyatt, R.J.; Martin, N.F., and Ciaranello, R.:* Catecholamine-related enzymes and normal personality variations (in preparation).

Dr. *R.J. Wyatt,* MD, Dr. *D.L. Murphy,* MD, and Dr. *R.H. Belmaker,* MD, Laboratory of Clinical Psychopharmacology, National Institute of Mental Health, Building 10, Room 4N206, *Bethesda, MD 20014* (USA)

Genetics and Psychopharmacology. Mod. Probl. Pharmacopsych., vol. 10, pp. 57–64,
ed. *J. Mendlewicz,* Brussels (Karger, Basel 1975)

Genetics of Monoamine Oxidase

D.S. Robinson and A. Nies

University of Vermont College of Medicine, Burlington, Vt., and
Dartmouth Medical School, Hanover, N.H.

The enzymes involved in the synthesis and degradation of the biogenic
amines have been widely investigated in man in recent years. Dopamine β-hy-
droxylase (DBH), catechol-O-methyltransferase (COMT) and monoamine oxidase (MAO) in particular have been studied in populations of normals and neuropsychiatric patients.

We have conducted ongoing studies of both patients and normals in connection with psychopharmacologic and biologic investigations of MAO activity
in psychiatric disorders. The goals of these investigations have been to determine
whether MAO activity measured in blood using a simple radioisotopic assay (23)
has clinical utility or biologic significance.

Platelet and plasma MAO activities were found to correlate with age, both in
normal subjects (24) and in depressed patients (18). Hindbrain MAO levels
assayed in *post mortem* specimens from patients who died from a variety of
causes also were found to correlate with age (25). These associations of MAO
activity with aging can be considered additional evidence relating altered amine
metabolism to such disorders as depression and parkinsonism whose incidence
increases with age. This is particularly true since it was also shown in the study
of human hindbrain that levels of at least one amine, norepinephrine, decrease
with age and inversely correlate with MAO activity (25). There is preliminary
evidence in man that COMT (1) and DBH (8) activities may also correlate
positively with age in certain tissues. Work in our laboratory using freshly
obtained *post mortem* tissue shows that the age-related changes in human brain
MAO activity are present in all of the individual areas of brain thus far studied (29).

Of equal interest are the questions whether or not other biologic factors
such as sex or genetic determinants might have a bearing on amine metabolism
or on psychopharmacologic responses. There are relatively few studies which
have addressed the question of genetic influences on response to psychopharma-

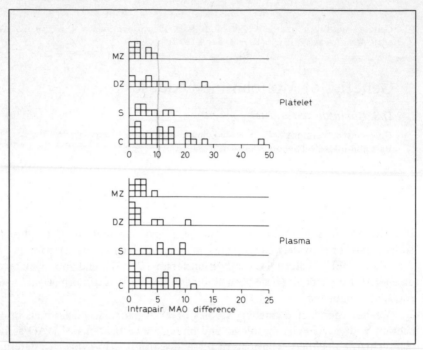

Fig. 1. Frequency histogram of intrapair differences in platelet monoamine oxidase (MAO) activity (nanomoles per milligram per hour) and plasma MAO activity (nanomoles per milliliter per hour) for monozygotic (MZ) twins (9 pairs), dizygotic (DZ) twins (11 pairs), same-sex siblings (S, 8 pairs) and age- and sex-matched controls (C, 20 pairs). MAO activities of platelets and plasma were measured using benzylamine as substrate by a previously described method (23).

cologic treatments. The existing studies will be discussed subsequently in this paper.

The epidemiologic evidence which shows an increasing incidence and prevalence of depression with aging also shows a marked preponderance of depressive illnesses in women. On examining our data for sex differences we found a statistically significant difference between men and women for platelet and plasma MAO activities with women having higher mean activities for the blood enzymes (24). In addition, women had higher mean hindbrain MAO activity than men, although this difference was not statistically significant (25). More recently *Murphy and Donnelly* (16) also reported higher platelet MAO activities in women using tryptamine as substrate.

Evidence for genetic control of MAO activity in man has been provided by 2 groups of investigators using the twin method (17, 34). *Wyatt et al.* using tryptamine as a substrate investigated platelet MAO activities as a possible biologic

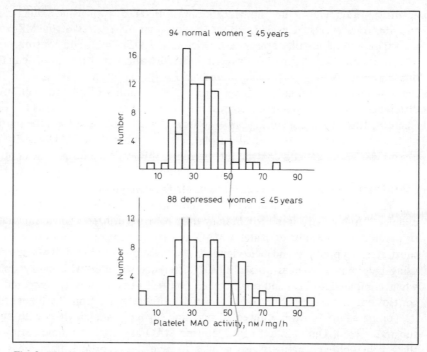

Fig. 2. Distribution of platelet MAO activities, expressed as nanomoles of benzylamine oxidized per milligram of protein per hour, for 94 normal women (upper histogram) and 88 depressed female outpatients under 45 years of age (lower histogram). Platelet MAO activity was measured by a previously described method (23). (Reproduced from *Robinson et al.,* 28, with permission of Excerpta Medica Foundation.)

marker for schizophrenia since various family, twin and adoptive studies have indicated that this disorder is at least partially genetically transmitted (11, 30). They found a high correlation of MAO activity between members of pairs of monozygotic (MZ) twins discordant for schizophrenia (r = 0.67) and normal MZ twin pairs (r = 0.94). In addition, platelet MAO activity in both members of the twin pairs discordant for schizophrenia was reduced when compared to the normal twins. The latter findings confirmed a previous study in which they reported platelet MAO values for 33 schizophrenic patients to be significantly lower than controls (15).

A similar approach to the study of the genetic control of MAO activity in man using the twin method has been carried out in our laboratory (17). These studies showed that genetic factors influence plasma and platelet MAO activities as measured with either of 2 substrates, benzylamine and tryptamine. Figure 1 shows the distributions of the intrapair differences in platelet and plasma MAO activities using benzylamine for MZ and dizygotic (DZ) twin pairs, sibling pairs and control subjects. It is evident that the intrapair differences of the MZ pairs are small, and all distribute near zero whereas the DZ, sibling and control intra-pair differences are larger and have a wider distribution. Also the calculated intraclass correlation coefficients were high for MZ twins, intermediate for DZ twins and sibling pairs and low for controls. The variability of the intrapair MAO differences of the MZ pairs was significantly less than the other groups (17, 18). There is, thus, quite convincing evidence from these studies that both the partic-ulate mitochondrial MAO activity of platelets and the soluble MAO activity of plasma are under genetic control. Furthermore, this evidence for genetic control of MAO with more than one substrate is of interest in light of the problems and controversies surrounding the existence of MAO isoenzymes.

The work of *Murphy and Wyatt* (15) mentioned above which reports lower platelet MAO activity in schizophrenics than controls utilized a single substrate, tryptamine. In a study of platelet MAO activity of schizophrenics using the 2 substrates, tryptamine and benzylamine, we have found reduced MAO activity using tryptamine whereas no significant difference was seen with benzylamine when compared to age- and sex-matched controls (18). However, compared to control brains the hippocampal MAO activity of the brains from 3 schizophren-ics compared to controls showed if anything higher MAO activities with both substrates (18). Our failure to find reduced MAO activities in limbic cortex of these schizophrenic patients also applies to several subcortical brain areas we have examined as well. The biologic or clinical significance of these findings, especially in connection with the genetic basis for schizophrenia, is presently unclear although *Wyatt et al.* (34) suggest that reduced platelet MAO activity may provide a genetic marker for vulnerability to schizophrenia. If our limited findings of brain MAO activity of schizophrenics is borne out in a larger series, it would appear that reduced MAO activity in schizophrenia may not generally apply to neural tissues. An explanation for enzymatic differences between tis-sues can be found in the probable occurrence of multiple forms of MAO with varying expressions from tissue to tissue.

Human populations can be examined for evidence of genetic heterogeneity by examining distributions of enzyme activities. We have analyzed the distribu-tions of MAO activity in populations of normals and depressives obtained during the course of our studies of the treatment of patients with MAO inhibitors (MAOI). Because of the established sex and age differences in platelet MAO activity, with the latter being particularly prominent in the older decades, our initial analysis was confined to women under 45 years of age. The distributions in both normals and a group of 88 depressed women under 45 years of age (fig. 2) can be seen to be continuous and is thus compatible with a polygenically controlled mode of inheritance of enzyme activity. However, the possibility of inheritence due to a single genetic factor cannot be excluded. The centers of distribution of the 2 populations are close, and although both are skewed to the right, the degree of skewness is greater for the depressed women than for the normals (fig. 2). This raises the possibility of the existence of a subgroup of depressed women with high MAO activity (> 52 nM/mg/h).

The relatively small sample led us to expand the analysis to include all female outpatients, a final sample of 104 women. The patient groups above and below the cutoff of 52 nM/mg/h were examined for differences in clinical characteristics. The 2 groups did not differ with respect to age or to type of depressive illness as assessed by clinical diagnosis and to degree of 'endogenicity' as assessed by numerical placement along a reactive-endogenous continuum (19, 26). However, the high MAO group did have significantly higher severity scores on several items of our standardized Hamilton interview such as depressed mood, guilt, impaired work and interest, situational anxiety and composite symptom scales measuring depression and psychic anxiety. When the analysis was further extended to include all depressed patients (men and women, inpatients and outpatients) assessed over the past 5 years with the standardized Hamilton interview and MAO determinations, the high MAO group (> 52 nM/mg/h) was again found to have higher Hamilton item scores in a similar pattern (28).

An interesting feature of this analysis was the fact that those female patients with high MAO activity who had been treated with phenelzine (60 mg/day) in a series of controlled clinical trials responded less well to MAOI therapy than a corresponding group with lower MAO activity also receiving phenelzine in the same dosage. Further work will be necessary to establish that high platelet MAO activity in depression is a genetic marker. If, in turn, it predicts nonresponsiveness to MAOI treatment, this would be of obvious pharmacogenetic interest.

There have been relatively few studies which have addressed the question of genetic factors determining response to psychopharmacologic treatments in affective disorders. Genetic control of tricyclic antidepressant drug metabolism has been demonstrated (2, 4). Therefore, it is conceivable that the response to treatment could have a genetic basis although the relationship of tricyclic blood levels to treatment outcome continues to be controversial (5–7, 12, 22). Because acetylator phenotype is a genetically determined trait, the recent reports of a relationship between therapeutic response to phenelzine and acetylator status are of great interest (10).

Angst (3) and *Pare and Mack* (20) have compared the response of first-degree relatives and the index patient to antidepressant drug therapy. Their findings have been interpreted to suggest that there is an intrafamily consistency of response to class of antidepressant drug. These studies provide suggestive clinical evidence that genetic factors influence response to the class of antidepressant drug. It is admittedly very difficult to carry out the type of prospective family studies which would be necessary to conclusively establish a familial coincidence of antidepressant responsiveness or nonresponsiveness. Nonetheless, such an undertaking employing controlled methods such as blind evaluation, prospectively chosen objective measures of change and careful classification and characterization of the patient population will be required to provide unequivocal evidence of familial and, therefore, likely genetic control of treatment response.

There is a sizable literature on the genetics of affective disorder using *Leonhard*'s (13) bipolar vs. unipolar distinction (9, 21, 32, 33). There is no work relating the genetics of these illnesses to the genetics of MAO activity although there is the report of *Murphy and Weiss* (14) showing reduced platelet MAO activity in bipolar depression and increased MAO activity in unipolar depression.

The genetics of neurotic depression are relatively unstudied although there is one study which reports that the expectency of affective disorders may be higher among relatives of such patients (31). This is of possible interest since our recent reports and review of the literature suggest that the MAOI drugs are most effective in neurotic, atypical or nonendogenous depressive illnesses (19, 26). Family studies of morbidity risk for affective disorders combined with determinations of enzyme levels and their relationships to outcome of antidepressant treatments offer opportunities for advancing our knowledge of these disorders and the possibility of improving treatment.

One genetically controlled factor which may influence the response to antidepressant treatment is sex. In our studies of the treatment of atypical and reactive depressions with the MAOI, phenelzine, we have found a sex difference in response. In 2 controlled trials the improvement shown by men was significantly greater than women ($p = 0.01$) as evaluated by a global improvement measure. The men also showed significantly greater improvement on individual symptom measures obtained from the standardized Hamilton interview (28).

It is apparent from this brief review that although there has been little investigation of the enzymes involved in biogenic amine metabolism, MAO has thus far received most study. There is an obvious need for further studies which would attempt to relate genetic control of enzyme activities to the familial occurrence of the affective disorders. Similarly, the pharmacogenetic aspects of MAOI drug therapy in these disorders also await further exploration.

Summary

Evidence for the genetic control of human MAO is now well established. The relationships of MAO activities to neuropsychiatric disorders or response to psychopharmacologic treatments are relatively unstudied. Preliminary findings from our own studies suggest that (1) blood MAO activity is a polygenically controlled trait; (2) there may be a subgroup of depressed patients with high MAO activity who are more severe symptomatically and more resistant to treatment, and (3) that men with atypical and mixed depressions respond more favorably than women to treatment with an MAO inhibitory drug.

Acknowledgements

The support of Public Health Service Grants 1 RO1 MH15533, 5 SO1 RR-05429 and TO2 05935 and awards from the Burroughs Wellcome Fund, Research Triangle Park, N.C., the Pharmaceutical Manufacturers Association Foundation, Washington, D.C., and the Warner-Lambert Charitable Foundation, Morris Plains, N.J., are acknowledged.

Dr. *Robinson* is a Burroughs Wellcome Fund Scholar in clinical pharmacology.

References

1 *Agathopoulos, A.; Nicolopoulos, D.; Matsaniotis, N., and Papadatos, C.:* Biochemical changes of catechol-*o*-methyltransferance during development of human liver. Pediatrics *47:* 125–128 (1971).

2 *Alexanderson, B.; Evans, D.A.P., and Sjoquist, F.:* Steady-state plasma levels of nortriptyline in twins. Influence of genetic factors and drug therapy. Brit. med. J. *iv:* 764–768 (1969).

3 *Angst, J.:* A clinical analysis of the effects of tofranil in depression. Longitudinal and followup studies. Treatment of blood relations. Psychopharmacologia, Berl. *2:* 381–407 (1961).

4 *Asberg, M.; Evans, D.A.P., and Sjoquist, F.:* Genetic control of nortriptyline plasma levels in man. J. med. Genet. *8:* 129–135 (1971).

5 *Asberg, M.; Cronholm, B.; Sjoquist, F., and Tuck, D.:* Relationship between plasma level and therapeutic effect of nortriptyline. Brit. med. J. *113:* 331–334 (1971).

6 *Braithwaite, R.A.; Goulding, R.; Theano, G.; Bailey, J., and Coppen, A.:* Plasma concentration of amitriptyline and clinical response. Lancet *i:* 1297–1300 (1972).

7 *Burrows, G.D.; Davies, B., and Scoggins, B.A.:* Plasma concentration of nortriptyline and clinical response in depressive illness. Lancet *112:* 619–623 (1972).

8 *Freedman, L.S.; Ohuchi, T.; Goldstein, M.; Axelrod, F.; Fish, I., and Dancis, J.:* Changes in human serum dopamine β-hydroxylase activity with age. Nature, Lond. *236:* 310, 311 (1972).

9 *Hopkinson, G.:* A genetic study of affective illness in patients over 50. Brit. J. Psychiat. *110:* 244–254 (1964).

10 *Johnstone, E.C. and Marsh, W.:* Acetylator status and response to phenelzine in depressed patients. Lancet *i:* 567–570 (1973).

11 *Kety, S.; Rosenthal, D.; Wender, B., and Schulsinger, F.:* The transmission of schizophrenia, pp. 345–362 (Pergamon, New York 1968).

12 *Kragh-Sorenson, P.; Asberg, M., and Eggert-Hansen, C.:* Plasma-nortriptyline levels in endogenous depression. Lancet *i:* 113–118 (1973).

13 *Leonhard, K.:* Aufteilung der endogenic Psychosen, 2nd ed. (Akademic Verlag, Berlin 1959).

14 *Murphy, D.L. and Weiss, R.:* Reduced monoamine oxidase activity in blood platelets from bipolar depressed patients. Amer. J. Psychiat. *128:* 1351–1357 (1972).

15 *Murphy, D.L. and Wyatt, R.J.:* Reduced monoamine oxidase activity in blood platelets from schizophrenic patients. Nature, Lond. *238:* 225, 226 (1972).

16 *Murphy, D.L. and Donnelly, C.H.:* Monoamine oxidase in man. Enzyme characteristics in human platelets, plasma, and other human tissues; in *Usdin* Neuropsychopharmacology of monoamines and their regulatory enzymes. Advances in biochemical psychopharmacology, vol. 12 (Raven Press, New York 1974).

17 *Nies, A.; Robinson, D.S.; Lamborn, K.R., and Lampert, R.:* Genetic control of platelet and plasma monoamine oxidase activity. Arch. gen. Psychiat. *28:* 834–838 (1973).

18 *Nies, A.; Robinson, D.S.; Harris, L.S., and Lamborn, K.R.:* Comparison of monoamine oxidase substrate activities in twins, schizophrenics, and controls; in *Usdin* Neuropsychopharmacology of monoamine and their regulatory enzymes. Advances in biochemical pharmacology, vol. 12 (Raven Press, New York 1974).

19 *Nies, A.; Robinson, D.S.; Ravaris, C.L., and Ives, J.O.:* The efficacy of the MAO inhibitor phenelzine. Dose effects and prediction of response. 9th Coll. Int. Neuropsychopharmacologicum, Paris 1974.

20 *Pare, C.M.B. and Mack, J.W.:* Differentiation of two genetically specific types of depression by the response to antidepressant drugs. J. med. Genet. *8:* 306–309 (1971).

21 *Perris, C.:* A study of bipolar (manic-depressive) and unipolar recurrent depressive psychoses. I. Genetic investigation. Acta psychiat. scand. *44:* suppl. 194, pp. 15–44 (1966).

22 *Rifkin, A.E.; Quitkin, F.M., and Klein, D.F.:* Plasma-nortriptyline levels in depression. Lancet *i:* 1258, 1259 (1973).

23 *Robinson, D.S.; Lovenberg, W.; Keiser, H., and Sjoerdsma, A.:* The effects of drugs in human blood platelet and plasma amine oxidase activity *in vitro* and *in vivo.* Biochem. Pharmacol. *17:* 109–119 (1968).

24 *Robinson, D.S.; Davis, J.M.; Nies, A.; Ravaris, C.L., and Sylwester, D.:* Relation of sex and aging to monoamine oxidase activity of human brain, plasma and platelets. Arch. gen. Psychiat. *24:* 536–539 (1971).

25 *Robinson, D.S.; Davis, J.M.; Nies, A.; Colburn, R.W.; Davis, J.N.; Bourne, H.R.; Bunney, W.E.; Shaw, D.M., and Coppen, A.J.:* Aging, monoamines, and monoamine-oxidase levels. Lancet *i:* 290, 291 (1972).

26 *Robinson, D.S.; Nies, A.; Ravaris, C.L., and Lamborn, K.R.:* The monoamine oxidase inhibitor, phenelzine, in the treatment of depressive-anxiety states. A controlled clinical trial. Arch. gen. Psychiat. *29:* 407–413 (1973).

27 *Robinson, D.S.; Nies, A.; Ravaris, C.L.; Ives, J.O., and Lamborn, K.R.:* Treatment response to MAO inhibitors. Relation to depressive typology and blood platelet MAO inhibition; in *Angst* Symp. Medicum Hoechst 8, Classification and Prediction of Outcome of Depression (in press).

28 *Robinson, D.S.; Nies, A.; Lamborn, K.R.; Ravaris, C.L., and Ives, J.O.:* Patterns of monoamine overdose activity in man. 9th Coll. Int. Neuropsychopharmacologicum, Paris 1974.

29 *Robinson, D.S.:* Changes in monoamine oxidase and monoamines with human development and aging. Fed. Proc. (in press).

30 *Rosenthal, D.; Wender, P.; Kety, S.; Schulsinger, J.; Welner, L., and Ostergaard, L.:* The transmission of schizophrenia, pp. 371–391 (Pergamon Press, New York 1968).

31 *Stenstedt, A.:* Genetics of neurotic depression. Acta psychiat. scand. *42:* 392–409 (1966).

32 *Winokur, G.; Cadoret; Dorzab, J., and Baker, M.:* Depressive disease. A genetic study. Arch. gen. Psychiat. *24:* 135–144 (1971).

33 *Woodruff, R.A.; Guze, S.B., and Clayton, P.J.:* Unipolar and bipolar primary affective disorder. Brit. J. Psychiat. *119:* 33–38 (1971).

34 *Wyatt, R.J.; Murphy, D.L.; Belmaker, R.; Cohen, S.; Donnelly, C.H., and Pollin, W.:* Reduced monoamine oxidase activity in platelets. A possible genetic marker for vulnerability to schizophrenia. Science *179:* 916–918 (1973).

Dr. *D.S. Robinson,* MD, and Dr. *A. Nies,* MD, University of Vermont College of Medicine, *Burlington, VT 05401* (USA)

Genetics and Psychopharmacology. Mod. Probl. Pharmacopsych., vol. 10, pp. 65–88, ed. *J. Mendlewicz*, Brussels (Karger, Basel 1975)

Monoamine Oxidase
Its Inhibition

Moussa B.H. Youdim

MRC Clinical Pharmacology Unit, and University Department of Clinical Pharmacology, Radcliffe Infirmary, Oxford

I. Introduction

The recognition of the central role of monoamine oxidase (MAO) (EC 1:4.3.4) in the disposition of pharmacologically active monoamines and the discovery of drugs that inhibit its action have stimulated much research. It was among the first of the monoamine-related enzymes to be discovered (46) and its reaction pathway described. Primary and secondary amines are oxidatively deaminated to the corresponding aldehyde, ammonia and hydrogen peroxide:

$$R - CH_2 - NH_2 + O_2 \rightarrow R - CH = CH + H_2O_2$$
$$R - CH = NH + H_2O \rightarrow R - CHO + NH_3.$$

However, in crude tissue preparations, catalase is present and hydrogen peroxide is broken down as follows:

$$H_2O_2 \rightarrow H_2O + \tfrac{1}{2}O_2,$$

the overall reaction being

$$R - CH_3 - NH_2 + \tfrac{1}{2}O_2 \rightarrow R - CHO + NH_3.$$

The functional role of MAO in the inactivation of putative neurotransmitter monoamines, in the de-toxification of other amines and the regulation of the free intra-neuronal amine concentration has been the subject of several reviews (27, 39, 40, 66, 112, 113, 119).

After some years of relative inactivity there has been an upsurge of interest in the functional role of MAO in the central nervous system and drugs that inhibit its activity. There are four basic areas of research which have had an influencing factor: (1) purification and characterisation of brain MAO; (2) overwhelming evidence for the presence of multiple molecular forms of MAO having different substrate and inhibitor specificities; (3) physiological regulation of MAO by steroid hormones, and (4) the advent of new drugs with 'selective' inhibition of multiple forms of MAO.

II. Basic Properties

In view of the widespread interest in the action of MAO it is desirable to review briefly some important physiochemical properties of this enzyme in the brain. Sub-cellular fractionation of neural tissue has revealed that almost all MAO activity is associated with the mitochondrion and is located in its outer membrane (95, 113, 126). About 10 % of this activity is intra-neuronal (32, 109). MAO activity is not uniformly distributed in the central nervous system. In the brain the highest activities are observed in the hypothalamus and caudate nucleus and the lowest activity in the median cortex (24, 118a, 130, 134, 140). Solubilised and highly purified MAO is pale yellow in colour. It is now accepted that the MAO is a flavoprotein, containing $1 M$ of flavin adenine dinucleotide (FAD) as a cofactor and $8 M$ of sulphydryl groups per mole of enzyme (see 12, 113, 126 for reviews). The flavin being covalently bound to the enzyme through a cysteinyl to a 4 amino acid peptide (62, 98, 120). Whether the sulphydryl groups take part in the catalytic reaction of MAO or have a structural function is not known at the present, although evidence exists to support both theories (113, 126). Information about the role of a metal in the function of MAO is now accumulating. Studies of iron deficiency in rats (107, 108) and iron deficiency anaemia in man (20, 141) have implicated the requirement of iron for full enzymatic activity. Whether iron functions as a cofactor or as part of the enzyme protein, or is required for the synthesis of MAO protein is not clear; however, it is evident from recent *in vivo* studies (107) that iron may very well play an important role in determining the activity of this enzyme and metabolism of biogenic amines in the body. Many membrane-bound enzymes, of which MAO is one, are thought to depend on the associated phospholipid for their functional as well as conformational stability. Liver MAO has an extremely high affinity for cardiolipin (77). When denuded of this lipid the enzyme becomes very unstable (79).

The methods available at the present to bring about the solubilisation of MAO are rather vigorous and harsh (31, 77, 78, 110, 136). They include treatment of the mitochondria with ultrasonic oscillation, the use of non-ionic and ionic detergents and extraction with organic solvents. A controversy has arisen as to whether the properties of solubilised and active form of the enzyme observed *in vitro* represent those *in vivo*, where the conditions may be very different (22,

54). Thus, the suggestion has been made that studying the enzyme in its more intimate environment would yield pertinent information regarding its physiological function.

III. Nature and Location of Multiple Forms of MAO

There are numerous reports that mitochondrial MAO in the peripheral tissue as well as in the central nervous system exists in more than one form (37, 38, 89, 123, 126, 127). Attempts have been made to separate amine oxidases which differ with regard to substrate and inhibitor specificities. These attempts have followed a number of basic approaches, electrophoretic separation of solubilised mitochondrial MAO into a number of active enzyme band on polyacrylamide gel having different substrate and inhibitor specificities (see 89 for review), the use of selective inhibitors (53, 56, 60, 61, 106, 135), induction of antibody to purified enzyme preparation (48, 70, 132), histochemical studies (44) and kinetic studies (45, 55–57). Although all techniques have met with some success in demonstrating the presence of more than one form of MAO, the results have not been universally accepted (54). Objections have been raised that the results of electrophoretic separation of MAO may stem from artifacts of solubilisation and purification procedures (22, 54), since these methods are rather harsh and vigorous. The suggestion has been made that multiple forms of MAO might arise from binding of different amounts or types of lipid material to a single enzyme species, thus conferring allotopic properties upon it (111, 115, 124, 132). Furthermore, the results of selective inhibition of MAO by drugs could be explained on the basis that either inhibitor active-enzyme complexes are formed or that the enzyme possesses more than one active site (1, 135).

No adequate explanation has been put forward as to the basis and the nature of MAO multiplicity, although polymerisation of solubilised basic active subunit (36), conformational changes (24, 131) and attachment to membrane material and phospholipid, thus conferring allotopic properties (111, 114, 115, 124), have been implicated. The presence of MAO attached to different population of mitochondria was first envisaged by *Youdim et al.* (137). Recent observations of *Kroon and Veldstra* (69), *Youdim* (125) and *Yang and Neff* (122) suggest that this may indeed be so. In the light of the above criticism, in a recent study (127) special care was taken to study brain MAO activity in the mitochondria which were not altered or damaged and were physiologically active. This investigation demonstrated that brain mitochondria are heterogenous with regards to MAO, succinate dehydrogenase and NADH-dehydrogenase. Furthermore, there exists a mitochondrial 'tyramine MAO' which is different from that of a 'dopamine MAO' and '5-hydroxytryptamine MAO', the latter enzymes being associated with mitochondria of the synaptosomes.

The differences in MAO activity may reflect the fact that brain mitochondria are not homogenous; thus, multiple forms of solubilised MAO may result from different populations of mitochondria (130a). Recent observations (122) have shown that disruption of mitochondria does not influence the ratio of the rates of monoamine deamination by MAO when compared with intact mitochondria.

The present finding does not allow any conclusions to be drawn as to whether the multiple forms of MAO arise from different proteins or one enzyme existing in different environments (allotopic properties) (114). These findings in no way diminish the underlying physiological significance of the various mitochondrial forms of MAO and may go some way to support their existence *in vivo*. There is no obvious correlation between heterogeneity of mitochondrial MAO and the electrophoretically separable solubilised multiple forms of this enzyme (134). The results, however, have shown that this enzyme has different distribution and activity in brain mitochondria (69, 122, 125, 127) and mitochondria can be separated mainly on the basis of size. It is possible that the mitochondrial MAO heterogeneity may result from microsomal contamination during homogenisation and centrifugation procedures; however, this is ruled out because no extra-mitochondrial MAO has been observed by electron-microscope histochemical studies (15). Because of the above findings it cannot be assumed that all mitochondrial MAO in one organ will (1) respond to the action of steroid hormones to the same extent with different substrates; (2) develop at the same rate in that or other organs, or (3) will be inhibited to the same extent by drugs (138).

All indications are that there are at least two distinct protein forms of MAO (70, 132) with different catalytic properties. Each form may exist in different states or environments. Evidence for the existence of multiple forms of mitochondrial MAO in the liver and brain is becoming overwhelming, although absolute proof of their occurrence *in vivo* will be difficult to obtain. However, the immunological experiments described originally by *Hartman* (47, 49) provide strong evidence that their *in vivo* existence is a reality. And recently *McCauley and Racker* (70) and *Youdim and Collins* (132) have reported the immunochemical separation of 2 enzymes from beef and rat brain, respectively, obtaining 2 immunoprecipitins, both enzymatically active but with different substrate and inhibitor specificities. Whether these forms can be further separated electro-phoretically has yet to be demonstrated. It is of interest that *Youdim and Collins* (132) and *Diaz Borges and D'Iorio* (28) have described the electrophoretic separation of MAO preparation into 2 fractions, one anodic form capable of oxidising tyramine and the other cathodic form dopamine or 5-hydroxytryptamine. The implications of 2 forms of MAO activity responsible for the oxidation of biologically active monoamines may represent some unknown complex system for controlling the rates of oxidation of these amines in the central nervous system.

IV. MAO Inhibitors

In studying the metabolism of arakylamines, tyramine and benzylamine, *Severina and Gorkin* (96) were able to selectively inhibit the oxidative deamination of the 2 amines. The kinetic studies on the inhibition of the oxidation of 5-hydroxytryptamine and tyramine by rat liver mitochondria (45) revealed that the 2 substrates are probably oxidised by two different MAO. The activity versus pH curves of MAO in the presence of hydrazine and non-hydrazine inhibitors suggested the presence of 2 systems capable of metabolising kynuramine but not equally sensitive to iproniazid, phenelzine, pargyline and tranylcypromine (135). When studying the pH activity curve with increasing concentrations of tranylcypromine and phenelzine, a second maximum was observed at lower pH levels. Similar results were obtained with the partially heat-inactivated rat liver mitochondrial enzyme preparations. It was, thus, concluded that the two pH maxima could be explained on the basis of (1) 2 distinct enzyme systems being present as a mixture; (2) active-enzyme-substrate complexes are formed, and (3) a unitory enzyme possessing more than one active site.

The first possibility was favoured by the findings with selective enzyme inhibition by drugs (135). Solubilisation of rat liver mitochondrial MAO revealed that this enzyme could be separated into a number of active forms with the technique of gel-electrophoresis (89). With the view that multiple forms of MAO having different substrate and inhibitor specificities may be a reality, drugs having selective inhibitory properties were looked for. Such studies of selective inhibition have recently gained momentum with the advent of some new drugs with this property, particularly clorgyline (MαB 9302) (42, 43, 61), deprenil (E-250) (64, 65) and N-cyclophenoxyethylamines (34, 45).

These inhibitors have one property in common: plotting percentage inhibition against log inhibitor concentration does not produce a single sigmoid curve (as observed, for example, with iproniazid or tranylcypromine), but rather a pair of sigmoid curves joined by a horizontal section where the inhibition is invariant. This pattern has been attributed to the presence of 2 forms of of the enzyme termed 'type A' and 'type B' (24, 42, 43, 53, 61, 75). Type A is sensitive to clorgyline and oxidatively deaminates 5-hydroxytryptamine, adrenaline, noradrenaline, tyramine and dopamine (24, 42, 43, 53, 61, 75). Type B, which is more resistant to clorgyline, oxidises phenylethylamine, benzylamine and tryptamine as well as tyramine and dopamine (fig. 1, 2), but not 5-hydroxytryptamine. Deprenil (E-250) has properties similar to clorgyline but with opposite effects, i.e. it inhibits 'type B' enzyme but is insensitive towards 'type A'. Whether these forms can be separated electrophoretically has yet to be fully demonstrated, although recent studies (28, 130a, 138) indicate that it may indeed be possible. Electrophoretically separated multiple forms of MAO have varying sensitivities to clorgyline (134, 138). Lipid environment of

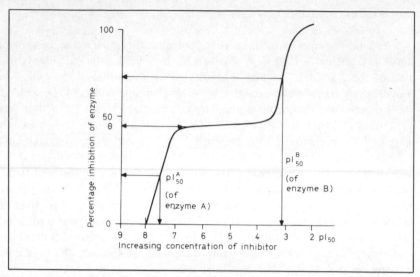

Fig. 1. Theoretical figure showing clorgyline type inhibition curve *in vitro*. Similar curve is also obtained *in vivo* (61).

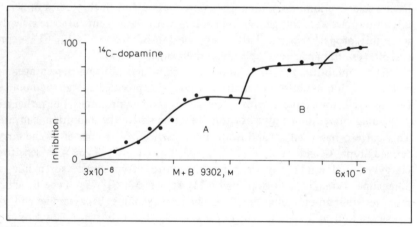

Fig. 2. The inhibition of whole human brain mitochondrial monoamine oxidase (MAO) by clorgyline (M & B 9302). The enzyme preparation was incubated with the inhibitor for 20 min at 37 °C before the addition of the substrate (^{14}C-dopamine) to a final concentration of 6.8×10^{-4} *M*. The results are expressed as percentage inhibition of the control enzyme activity. A and B represent a mixture of 2 enzymes. When tyramine was the substrate a similar curve was obtained. However, with kynuramine as substrate a normal sigmoidal dose response curve was obtained at the position of enzyme B.

MAO is thought to play an important role in its specificity (54, 111, 115, 124) and multiplicity. Multiple forms of rat liver mitochondrial and cat brain mitochondrial MAO as separated by gel-electrophoresis have varying phospholipid content (111, 134, 138). The forms with least phospholipid material appear to be more resistant to inhibition by clorgyline (type B enzyme) (132, 134, 138). In this context it is interesting to note that treatment of rat liver mitochondria with chaotropic agents (which removes substantial amounts of phospholipid) renders the enzyme insensitive to clorgyline (54, 114), thus abolishing type A enzyme activity (54, 114). The evidence from electrophoretic studies of soluble mitochondrial MAO which reveals multiple forms in the different tissues would now seem to be better interpreted on the basis of recent data (28, 70, 132, 133) as probably representing 2 distinct enzyme forms.

V. Inhibition of MAO in Human Brain

It is now 22 years since the discovery of iproniazid as a potent inhibitor of MAO and 17 years since its introduction as an anti-depressant. Since then a large number of new MAO inhibitor anti-depressants has been developed and introduced for therapeutic usage. Although there remain unsolved questions as to therapeutic efficacy and toxicity, the trend of recent clinical investigation and therapeutic experience affirms that MAO inhibitor anti-depressant effects occur in significant proportions of depressed patients (2, 63). MAO inhibitors have been widely used in the treatment of depressive illness, and it has been tacitly accepted that their beneficial effect stems from inhibition of MAO alone and the resulting elevation of monoamine concentrations in the central nervous system (83). There had previously been no convincing explanation as to why some drug inhibitions of the enzyme are effective in the treatment of depression and others are not. The question has been raised as to whether their anti-depressant clinical effects can be attributed entirely to inhibition of MAO, since most of these drugs have a variety of additional pharmacological effects, including the inhibition of amine re-uptake after post-synaptic release (29, 50). It would now seem reasonable to suggest that the answer lies in terms of differential inhibition of multiple forms of MAO. This hypothesis brings in its train an important corollary: if it were to be proved correct, it follows that the synthesis of specific inhibitors tailored either to an individual form of the enzyme at a particular site in the central nervous system or tailored to its substrate should be within our grasp. Implicit in this argument is the conclusion that the therapeutic effectiveness of MAO inhibitors relies on a localised accumulation of a particular amine substrate at a specific site in the brain. It has been shown that the substrate and inhibitor specificities of rat and human liver and brain differ (see 89 for review). For example, rat and human liver and brain MAO form 1 de-

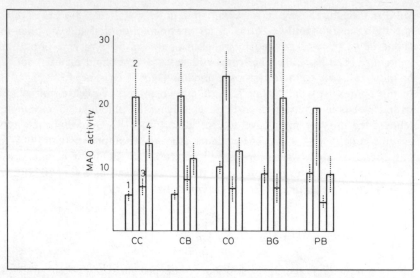

Fig. 3. Distribution of human brain mitochondrial MAO (mean ± SEM) in different anatomical areas brain from 10 untreated (control) subjects. Substrates: 1 = kynuramine; 2 = tyramine; 3 = tryptamine; 4 = dopamine. Anatomical areas: CC = cerebral cortex; CB = cerebellum; CO = centrum ovale; BG = basal ganglia; PB = pineal body. Abbreviations same throughout.

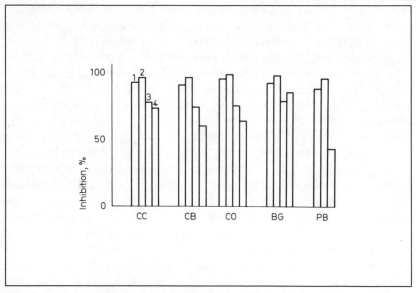

Fig. 4. Mitochondrial MAO activity in brain from human subjects after treatment with Marplan (isocarboxazid). The results are the means of 12 brains.

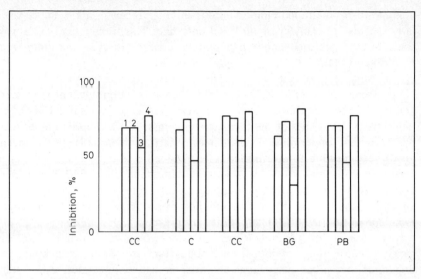

Fig. 5. Mitochondrial MAO activity in brains from subjects after treatment with Parnate (tranylcypromine). For details see figure 4. The results are mean of 12 brains.

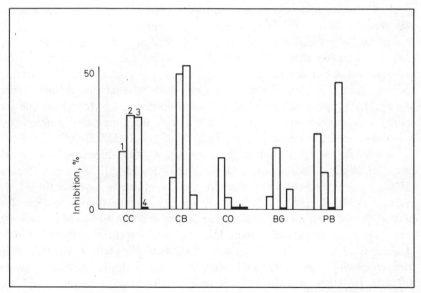

Fig. 6. Mitochondrial MAO activity in brains from human subjects after treatment with clorgyline (M & B 9302). For details see figure 4. The results are means of 13 brains.

aminates tyramine much more rapidly than MAO forms 4 and 5 and is particularly sensitive to tranylcypromine and portyline. This finding may explain why some MAO inhibitors induce hypertensive crises with tyramine more readily than others (71).

To suggest a possible biochemical basis for a tranylcypromine-cheese interaction from such data is relatively straightforward. The problem of the differing abilities of MAO inhibitors to alleviate depression is not as clear-cut, if one is to judge from the results of the recent experiments. MAO inibitors are useful for the treatment of terminal depression in geriatric subjects (9). It has recently (140) been possible to investigate brains obtained at autopsy from such patients treated with tranylcypromine (Parnate), clorgyline (MαB 9302) and isocarboxazid (Marplan) and from untreated controls from the same hospital, whose enzyme activity and distribution did not differ from previously investigated non-depression brains (24) (fig. 3). In each group whole mitochondrial MAO activity was measured in cerebral cortes, cerebellum, centrum ovale, basal ganglia, pineal body, hypothalamus, brain stem and pons using kynuramine dopamine, tyramine, tryptamine and dopamine as substrates. After tranylcypromine, the oxidation of tryptamine was inhibited less than that of the other substrates and dopamine oxidation was the most effectively inhibited substrate in all areas examined (fig. 4). With isocarboxazid dopamine oxidation was least affected. In the pineal body, in fact, the rate of dopamine oxidation was similar to that of untreated brain, whereas the oxidation of tyramine was completely blocked (fig. 5). After clorgyline (fig. 6) complex pattern of enzyme inhibition was seen; in the pineal body, basal ganglia and centrum ovale oxidation of tryptamine was unaffected, whereas inhibition of enzyme from the cerebral cortex was greater than 50 %. Similarly, dopamine oxidation was normal in the cerebral cortex but decreased to almost half in the pineal body. It is interesting to note that *Neff and Goridis* (75) have reported that pineal body contains mainly MAO type A as identified by inhibition curves by clorgyline. The above results from human brain studies confirm this, suggesting that pineal MAO is sensitive to inhibition by clorgyline (fig. 6), i.e., type A MAO.

Evidence has been obtained *in vitro* and *in vivo* suggesting that multiple forms of MAO of human, rat and cat brain (24, 134, 137) do indeed possess differing sensitivities to clorgyline. *In vivo* experiments have confirmed these findings (134). Recent studies have shown that the situation of multiple forms of MAO to be even more complex than it was thought to be (56). *In vivo* they may work as an integrated system. Many more observations with brain obtained at autopsy from patients treated with MAO inhibitors will be needed before a firm conclusion can be reached. However, such autopsy specimens are very difficult to come by. Some investigators have overcome this problem by studying the platelet MAO activity of patients treated with MAO inhibitors with the implications that it may reflect brain MAO activity (73, 74, 88, 121). Objections have been raised that the platelet MAO may not be representative of the enzyme activity in the central nervous system (128). All indications are that the platelet MAO is of 'type B' enzyme described previously in this chapter. More careful studies in humans using the platelet MAO as a peripheral marker and different MAO inhibitor anti-depressants are badly needed.

VI. Physiology of MAO in the Central Nervous System

It is recognised that MAO plays an important role in the degradation of biologically active monoamines in the central and peripheral tissues (9, 14, 24, 66, 91, 118, 137). The biogenic amines are stored in an inactive form in the sub-cellular particles (amine storage granules) of nervous tissue. Such amines can be released into the circulation either by nerve stimulation or by pharmacological agents and could cause pharmacological effects which might be drastic if the excess is not metabolised. Possibly it is for this reason that an enzyme such as MAO capable of metabolising the amines is provided. The enzyme is present both in the extra-neuronal as well as in the intra-neuronal tissue. Over the years a large body of evidence has accrued pointing to changes in monoamine metabolism in mental illnesses characterised by alteration in mood (5, 9, 18, 26, 71, 80). Perhaps the most important set of observations in this area concerns the property which MAO inhibiting drugs possess, of bringing about at lightening effect in depressed patients (2, 63, 81, 82, 92). Whilst it has not occurred to most authors to question that, the action results solely from the ability of these compounds to inhibit MAO, thereby raising the level of neurotransmitter at specific sites in the central nervous system, The fact remains that the anti-depressive effect is not shared to an equal extent by all drugs in the groups (89). An attempt has been made by one school to explain this puzzling finding in terms of differing ability of MAO inhibiting drugs to prevent amine re-uptake (50); however, it has seemed that an explanation might better be sought in terms of differential inhibitory capacity of these drugs on the multiple forms of MAO in human brain (24, 89, 90, 140). The suggestion has been made that these drugs have the property of distinguishing between different forms of MAO which are present in the mitochondria of the central nervous system (90, 122, 137, 140).

There have been many hypotheses as to the role MAO plays in the detoxification of amines. *Blaschko* (10a) finds fault with the suggestion (142) that MAO is responsible for the de-toxification of high concentrations of amines of bacterial origin in the intestine. He has pointed out that it is very unlikely for the amine concentration to be so high as to require the amount of enzyme actually present. A 'hypertensive crisis' in depressed patients due to the interaction of cheese and certain MAO inhibitors was first reported by *Blackwell* (10). This crisis occurs only with some inhibitors, such as tranylcypromine (Parnate) and substances related structurely to amphetamine. *Asatoor* (4) demonstrated that there is a large quantity of tyramine in certain cheeses. Under normal conditions the tyramine is oxidatively deaminated either in the intestine or after absorption, and that the substance which causes the 'hypertensive crisis' was tyramine (71). Until recently it had been customary to consider oxidative deamination as the only catabolic mechanism for tyramine and other monoamines such as dopamine and 5-hydroxytryptamine (serotonin). It appears that a second alternative catabolic pathway for oral and endogenous monoamines may exist via conjugation (72, 99, 139). When MAO is inhibited, it is likely that the conjugation pathway is capable of acting as a safety valve mechanism. A group of subjects exists within the population in whom this second pathway is defective (99, 139). This finding has at least one important implication for clinical practice. Patients being treated with MAO inhibiting drugs, normally possess conjugating enzymes, its absence in certain individuals might make such therapy dangerous for them. Recent studies (89) indicate that depressive patients who had manifested severe hypertensive reaction while on MAO inhibitory therapy are unable to conjugate oral tyramine to any large extent.

The gut has a high concentration of serotonin (5-hydroxytryptamine) and because of its implication in intestinal mobility, *Davison* (30) suggested that MAO is responsible for regulating the concentration of this amine. Interest in the role of MAO in the metabolism of brain serotonin has been stimulated by the findings that inhibitors of this enzyme can increase the level of amine in the brain (105) and implication of this amine in depressive illness. It is known that serotonin is a good substrate for MAO both *in vivo* and *in vitro* (11, 16, 17). It is of interest to note that *Bogdanski and Udenfriend* (17) have shown that the distribution of serotonin parallels that of MAO in the dog and cat brain, whereas the distribution of catacholamines and MAO in bovine adrenal medulla is different (13). Serotonin can be released from its bound form by administration of reserpine, thus making the amine available to MAO (19). Recent studies (102, 104, 116) have shown that MAO may play an important role in regulating the noradrenaline and serotonin content of sub-cellular particles. As serotonin is released by reserpine there is rapid depletion of the 'active' amine, and this has led *Brodie et al.* (116) to postulate that, just as cholinesterase is responsible for inactivating acetylcholine, MAO may play a similar role in destroying an excess of a neurohormonal transmitter such as serotonin. 5-hydroxytryptamine in the brain is synthesized from hydroxylation of tryptophan to 5-hydroxytryptophan, this amino acid is decarboxylated to 5-hydroxytryptamine. The 5-hydroxytryptamine which is synthesized is thought to be passed into one of two compartments; either into the storage granule pool or when that is fully saturated it spills over ('functional pool') and is principally oxidatively deaminated by intraneuronal MAO (76). It has been suggested the level of 'functional pool' of 5-hydroxytryptamine within the neuron is regulated by the availability of

5-hydroxytryptamine to MAO and granular re-uptake processes (39, 40). Deficiency of neuronal 5-hydroxytryptamine has been implicated in suicide and terminal depression (2, 5, 18, 26, 63, 80–82, 92). This finding is made more significant by the report of decreased 5-hydroxyindoleacetic acid, the oxidatively deaminated product of 5-hydroxytryptamine. It has been reported on a number of occasions that administration of tryptophan will potentiate the antidepressant effect of MAO inhibitors (25), thereby increasing the brain levels of 5-hydroxytryptamine (102). MAO inhibitors appear to have a considerably greater effect on 5-hydroxytryptamine containing neurons than on those containing catecholamines (104, 116).

The role of this enzyme in the metabolism of catecholamines is rather obscure. Both adrenaline and noradrenaline are good substrates for MAO *in vitro;* however, there has been some doubt whether MAO is the chief physiological inactivator of adrenaline and noradrenaline. Evidence supporting the inactivation of the catecholamines by MAO came from the work of *Schayer et al.* (93, 94). It was demonstrated that injected ^{14}C-adrenaline is metabolised by MAO in rats and its metabolites could be recovered in the urine. It was concluded, therefore, that MAO plays a role in the metabolism of adrenaline. An increase in the concentration of noradrenaline in the brain after inhibition of MAO was shown by *Shore et al.* (97). Evidence has been provided (3, 6, 33) that adrenaline, noradrenaline and dopamine are metabolised by O-methylation and could precede oxidative deamination by MAO. O-methylation is now known to be the major pathway of the metabolism of catecholamines. *Kopin* (67) demonstrated that about 25 % of adrenaline is deaminated while about 66 % is O-methylated by catechol O-methyl transferase. *Kopin and Axelrod* (68), examining the role of MAO in the metabolism of noradrenaline, presented evidence to indicate that to a large extent MAO plays a role in the metabolism of more firmly bound stores of noradrenaline as released by reserpine, whereas noradrenaline released in active form by nerve stimulation is not inactivated by MAO but by catechol O-methyl transferase. Furthermore, it was shown (41) that inhibition of MAO by iproniazid potentiates the response of the nictitating membrane to tryamine but not to adrenaline. This was one of the first important pieces of evidence that MAO did not act directly on the catecholamines under physiological conditions.

The re-uptake mechanism is now thought to be acting as a primary system of non-chemical inactivation of adrenaline and noradrenaline released at the receptor site (58, 59). The function of intra-neuronal MAO may, therefore, be to metabolise released neurotransmitter monoamines before or after re-uptake into the nerve endings. However, this process itself may depend on the state of MAO present in the nerve terminals (117). The re-uptake process appears to be governed by the relative concentration of free intra- and extra-neuronal amines. The results suggest that MAO is essential for keeping cytoplasmic levels of noradrenaline and 5-hydroxytryptamine in the neuron low. Under conditions when MAO is inhibited, the amine storage (uptake) capacity of granules which is limited, becomes gradually exhaused with time and the level of neuronal amine rises. Further support for the physiological importance of intra-neuronal MAO comes from the work of *Kroon and Veldstra* (69), and *Youdim* (63, 127). Their demonstration that brain mitochondria are heterogeneous with regard to MAO activity lends support to the functional role of this enzyme in the neurons. They have presented strong evidence for the presence of a 'dopamine MAO', 5-hydroxytryptamine MAO in the nerve ending particles (synaptosomes) differing from 'noradrenaline and tyramine deaminating synaptosomes'. The suggestion has been made that deamination of non-methylated biogenic monoamines can take place in the neurons.

VII. Regulation of MAO

There is now evidence available that intra-neuronal MAO plays an important part in regulation functionally active pools of monoamines in the central nervous system (39, 40). How this 'regulating' catabolism takes place is not known. However, it might be regulated either by induced alteration in MAO activity by steroids (138) or it is possible that each amine substrate in the neuron at level of pre-synaptic cytoplasma interacts with one or more of the multiple forms of MAO, thereby causing small but not readily reversible changes in conformation (allotopic changes) with a corresponding change or alteration of specific activity but not of affinity for the substrate. The interaction could occur either during the folding of the enzyme chain or, perhaps, during the catalytic process itself. We may, therefore, have a simple self-regulatory mechanism by which an increase in the intra-neuronal concentration of a particular amine is accompanied by the activation of a relatively specific form of MAO (24). This hypothesis has received some support from the rate of oxidation of dopamine in the uterus MAO (23), aorta MAO (103) and adrenal gland MAO (129), homogenates prepared from rats pre-treated for several days with pharmacological doses of dopamine precursor *L*-dopa (dihydroxy-phenylalanine). It is known that *L*-dopa does not alter protein synthesis. Let us consider the first possibility that naturally occurring steroids may affect MAO activity (138). Much information has accumulated on various aspects of neuro-endocrine functions during oestrous cycle of animals and pregnancy. The effects of hormones on release and metabolism of biogenic amines in adult animals of severals species are well documented (86, 100, 101, 126, 138). Variation in MAO activity using histochemical techniques was originally noted in human endometrium during the menstrual cycle (21), which was confirmed later by *Southgate et al.* (101). Changes in MAO activity during the oestrous cycle have been reported to occur in a number of organs, including the brains of rodents (52). Evidence is available that corti-costeroids and oestrogens inhibit catecholamine and indoleakylamine catab-olism, and progesterone stimulates this process *in vitro* as well as *in vivo* (52, 84, 85, 138). Because of the suggested link between MAO activity and ovarian steroid production rates (52), an indirect assessment of the changes in proges-terone production during the oestrous cycle of rat in the ovaries and adrenal glands contents has been made (52). It is apparent that the changes in MAO activity and progesterone content ran nearly parallel. It should be noted that in the adrenocorticoid tissue of the dog the bulk of progesterone was found in the true mitochondrial fraction in addition to the highest MAO activity (51). It has been suggested (138) that the observed changes in MAO activity during the oestrous cycle are the result of simultaneous changes in the blood concentration of progesterone (which stimulates) and oestrogens (which inhibit) MAO activity. However, since ovaries secreted a number of other central active progesterone derivatives, they could also be involved. The mechanism of action by which steroids alter MAO activity *in vivo* is not fully understood. However, steroids may exert their action on the outer mitochondrial membrane (where MAO resides) which leads to conformational (allotopic) modifications of its structure, thus affecting MAO activity (138). The lack of an immediate response to pro-gesterone *in vitro* may be due to the fact that the initial effect on membrane permeability is too small to be detected and the duration of the exposure to progesterone is too short. Similar changes have recently been confirmed for human platelet MAO (8).

The physiological significance of steroid-induced changes inMAO activity and amine metabolism is not fully understood. The extensive work of *Ball et al.* (7) on physico-chemical interaction between steroids and biogenic monoamines reflect an important additional action of these steroids hormones, since they may play a role in the regulation of the catabolism of monoamines as early studies indicate that amines and hormones may act as a single physiological unit (87).

VIII. Future Development

There are numerous drugs that are capable of inhibiting MAO and have been used in the treatment of depression; they fall into 2 groups, the hydrazines and the non-hydrazines. It is apparent from the studies reported in this chapter that they inhibit human brain MAO *in vivo* to a different degree depending on the substrate used to measure its activity. There is some question as to whether their anti-depressant efficacy is related entirely to inhibition of MAO and not to some other secondary effect. It is clear that although MAO could be fully inhibited using one substrate, e.g. tyramine, the use of a second substrate, e.g. dopamine, may not be. Therefore, the dosage and type of drug used and the heterogeneity of MAO may contribute significantly to the clinical efficacy of the MAO inhibitors. As regards to dosage their use has not been pushed into pharmacological levels with the different MAO inhibitors. In view of this we lack much information as to whether the patient has received sufficient drug to inhibit MAO activity fully. To monitor MAO activity by measuring urinary amines and their metabolites may give erroneous results. Platelet MAO has been used as a model reflecting brain MAO activity (73, 74). Although objections have been raised (128) a direct assessment of platelet MAO could be made if more than one substrate is employed to measure its activity. A number of observations have indicated fluctuation of MAO activity in animals and man related to the hormonal state. Is it possible that patients with depression have a higher MAO activity and may, therefore, need a relatively large dose of MAO inhibitors to produce therapeutic effect.

In 1969 (137) we offered an approach we thought in better accord with multiple forms of MAO and its inhibitors. It may be possible to correlate the therapeutic effect of these compounds with their inhibitory action on a particular form of the enzyme. With this in mind it was suggested (24) that an approach should be made in synthesis of specific selective inhibitors tailored either to an individual form of the enzyme or to the biogenic amines, thus eliminating some of the side-effects. With this in mind *Yang and Neff* (122) using the newly synthesized 'selective' inhibitors clorgyline and deprenil have been able to selectively inhibit the various forms of MAO and, thus, raise the levels of either the neurotransmitter 5-hydroxytryptamine or β-phenylethylamine. It is to be hoped that synthesis of specific MAO inhibitors directed at the active site of MAO will enhance the understanding of the role of this enzyme and may lead not only to the more effective treatment of depressive illness but also to an understanding of the underlying possible chemical lesion.

Summary

Some 50 years ago the enzyme MAO was discovered by *Hare* and in the early 1930s *Blaschko* suggested that MAO may play an important role in the catabolism of monoamines in the central nervous system. With the discovery of iproniazid as an inhibitor of MAO and its introduction as an anti-depressant, many aspects of MAO activity and biogenic amine metabolism in experimental animals and man were examined. Although many other inhibitors of MAO were discovered and used therapeutically as anti-depressants, these drugs fell into disrepute largely because of their side-effects. Furthermore, their anti-depressant properties were questioned. After some years of relative inactivity there is now a revival of interest in the functional role of MAO in the central nervous system and drugs that inhibit or stimulate its activity 'specifically'. The basic reason for the upsurge of interest is that the enzyme from many tissues, including the brain of animals as well as man, has been purified and characterised. The evidence that neuronal MAO exist with different substrate and inhibitor specificities has led to the suggestion that they have physiological function and that deamination of non-methylated biogenic monoamines can take place in neurons. These findings have led to the advent of new drugs (clorgyline and depranil) with 'selective' inhibition of enzyme forms. Their possible usage in the chemotherapy of depressive illness should be considered seriously. Fluctuation in peripheral organs as well as brain MAO is well documented. Recently they have been associated with changes in naturally occurring steroids. Although a decrease in platelet and brain MAO activity has been reported in a number of affect disorders (schizophrenia and biopolar depression) the results of these findings have recently been questioned (20, 141). Obviously further study in this area of research discussed is badly needed.

References

1 *Achee, F.M.; Togula, G., and Gabay, S.:* Studies of monoamine oxidase. Properties of the enzyme in bovine and rabbit brain mitochondria. J. Neurochem. *22:* 651–662 (1974).

2 *Angst, J.:* Symposium. Present status in research and clinical use of MAO inhibitors. Proc. 9th Int. Coll. Neuro-Psychopharmacology, Paris 1974.

3 *Armstrong, M.D.; McMillan, A., and Shaw, K.N.F.:* 3-Methoxy-4-hydroxy-*D*-mandelic acid. A urinary metabolite of norepinephrine. Biochem. biophys. acta *25:* 422–423 (1957).

4 *Asatoor, A.M.; Levi, A.J., and Milne, M.D.:* Hypertensive action by tyramine in cheese. Lancet *iii:* 733 (1963).

5 *Ashcrof, G.W.; Crawford, T.B.B.; Eccelston, D.; Sharman, D.F.; MacDougall, E.J.; Stanton, J.B., and Binns, J.K.:* 5-Hydroxyindole compounds in the cerebro-spinal fluid of patients with psychiatric or neurological diseases. Lancet *ii:* 1049–1052 (1966).

6 *Axelrod, J.:* O-methylation of epinephrine and other catechols *in vitro* and *in vivo.* Science *126:* 400–401 (1957).

7 *Ball, P.; Knuppen, M.; Houpt, H., and Breuer, H.:* Interactions between oestrogens and catecholamines and other catechols by the catechol-O-methyl transferase of human liver. J. clin. Endocrin. *34:* 736–746 (1972).

8 *Belmaker, R.H.; Murphy, D.L.; Wyatt, R.J., and Loriaux, L.D.:* Human platelet monoamine oxidase changes during the menstrual cycle. Personal commun. (1974).

9 *Bevan Jones, A.B.; Pare, C.M.B.; Nicholson, W.J.; Price, K., and Stacey, R.S.:* Brain amine concentration after monoamine oxidase inhibitor administration. Brit. med. J. *i:* 17–19 (1972).

10 *Blackwell, B.:* Hypertensive crisis due to monoamine oxidase inhibitors. Lancet *ii:* 849–851 (1963).

10a *Blaschko, H.:* Amine oxidase and amine metabolism. Pharmacol. Rev. *4:* 415–453 (1952).

11 *Blaschko, H.:* 5-hydroxytryptamine. pp. 50–57 (Pergamon Press, Oxford 1957).

12 *Blaschko, H.:* The natural history of amine oxidases. Rev. Physiol. Biochem. Pharmacol. *70:* 84−148 (1974).

13 *Blaschko, H.; Hagen, J.M., and Hagen, P.:* Mitochondrial enzymes and chromaffin granules. J. Physiol., Lond. *139:* 316−322 (1957).

14 *Bloom, F.E. and Giarman, N.J.:* Physiologic and pharmacologic consideration of biogenic amines in the nervous system. Annu. Rev. Pharmacol. *8:* 229−247 (1968).

15 *Boadle, M.C. and Bloom, F.E.:* A method for the fine structural localisation of monoamine oxidase. J. Histochem. Cytochem. *17:* 331−340 (1969).

16 *Bogdanski, D.F. and Udenfriend, S.:* Serotonin and monoamine oxidase in brain. J. Pharmacol. exp. Ther. *116:* 7−8 (1956).

17 *Bogdanski, D.F.; Weissbach, H., and Udenfriend, S.:* The distribution of serotonin, 5-hydroxytryptophan decarboxylase and monoamine oxidase in brain. J. Neurochem. *1:* 272−278 (1957).

18 *Bourne, H.R.; Bunney, W.E.; Colbourn, R.W.; Davis, J.M.; Davis, J.N.; Shaw, D.M., and Coppen, A.J.:* Noradrenaline, 5-hydroxytryptamine and 5-hydroxyindole acetic acid in hind brain of suicidal patients. Lancet *ii:* 805−808 (1968).

19 *Brodie, B.B.; Tomich, E.G.; Kuntzman, R., and Shore, P.A.:* On the mechanism of action of reserpine. Effect of reserpine on capacity of tissue to bind serotonin. J. Pharmacol. exp. Ther. *119:* 461−465 (1957).

20 *Callender, S.; Grahame-Smith, D.G.; Woods, H.F., and Youdim, M.B.H.:* Reduction of platelet monoamine oxidase activity in iron deficiency anaemia. Brit. J. Pharmacol. *52:* 447−448P (1974).

21 *Cohen, S.; Bitensky, L., and Chayen, J.:* The study of monoamine oxidase activity by histochemical procedures. Biochem. Pharmacol. *14:* 223−226 (1965).

22 *Collins, G.G.S.:* Summary of section I. Adv. biochem. Psychopharmacol. *5:* 129−132 (1972).

23 *Collins, G.G.S.; Pryse-Davies, J.; Sandler, M., and Southgate, J.:* Effect of pretreatment with estradiol and progesterone and DOPA on monoamine oxidase activity in the rat. Nature, Lond. *226:* 642−643 (1971).

24 *Collins, G.G.S.; Sandler, M.; Williams, E.D., and Youdim, M.B.H.:* Multiple forms of human brain mitochondrial monoamine oxidase. Nature, Lond. *225:* 817−820 (1970).

25 *Coppen, A.J.; Shaw, D.M., and Farrell, J.P.:* Potentiation of the antidepressive effect of a monoamine oxidase inhibitor by tryptophan. Lancet *i:* 79−81 (1963).

26 *Coppen, A.J.; Shaw, D.M.; Herzberg, B., and Maggs, R.:* Tryptophan in the treatment of depression. Lancet *ii:* 1178−1180 (1968).

27 *Costa, E. and Sandler, M.:* Monoamine oxidases. New vistas (Raven Press, New York 1972).

28 *Diaz Borges, J.M. and D'Iorio, A.:* Polyacrylamide gel electrophoresis of rat liver mitochondrial monoamine oxidase. Canad. J. Biochem. *51:* 1089−1095 (1973).

29 *Davis, J.M.:* Arch. gen. Psychiat. *13:* 552−569 (1965).

30 *Davison, A.N.:* Physiological role of monoamine oxidase. Physiol. Rev. *38:* 729−747 (1958).

31 *Erwin, V.G. and Hellerman, L.:* Mitochondrial monoamine oxidase. I. Purification and characterisation of bovine kidney enzyme. J. biol. Chem. *242:* 4230−4238 (1968).

32 *Fahn, S.; Rodman, J.S., and Cote, L.J.:* Association of tyrosine hydroxylase with synoptic vesicles in bovine condate nucleus. J. Neurochem. *16:* 1293−1300 (1969).

33 *Pellerin, J. and D'Iorio, A.:* Methylation of the 3-OH position of catechol acids by rat liver and kidney preparations. Canad. J. Biochem. *36:* 491−497 (1958).

34 *Fuller, R.W.:* Kinetic studies and *in vivo* effects of a new monoamine oxidase inhibitor,

N-2(O-chlorophenoxy-ethyl) cyclopropylamine. Biochem. Pharmacol. *17:* 2097–2106 (1968).

35 *Fuller, R.W.:* Selective inhibition of monoamine oxidase. Adv. biochem. Psycho-pharmacol. *5:* 339–354 (1972).

36 *Gomes, B.; Igane, I.; Kloepfer, H.G., and Yasunobu, K.T.:* Amine oxidase. XIV. Isolation and characterisation of the multiple beef amine oxidase components. Arch. Biochem. Biophys. *132:* 16–27 (1969).

37 *Gorkin, V.Z.:* Monoamine oxidase. Pharmacol. Rev. *18:* 115–120 (1966).

38 *Gorkin, V.Z.:* Monoamine oxidases. Versatility of catalytic properties and possible biological functions. Adv. Pharmacol. Chemother. *11:* 1–50 (1973).

39 *Grahame-Smith, D.G.:* How important is the synthesis of brain 5-hydroxytryptamine in the physiological control of its central function? Adv. Biochem. Psycho-pharmacol. *10:* 83–91 (1974).

40 *Green, A.R. and Grahame-Smith, D.G.:* 5-Hydroxytryptamine and other indoles in the central nervous system; in *Snyder, Iversen and Iversen* Handbook of psychopharmacology (Plenum Press, New York 1975).

41 *Griesemer, E.C.; Barsky, J.; Dragstedt, C.A.; Wells, J.A., and Zeller, E.A.:* Potentiating effect of iproniazid on the pharmacological action of sympathomimetic amine. Proc. Soc. exp. Biol. Med. *84:* 699–701 (1953).

42 *Hall, D.W.R. and Logan, B.W.:* Further studies on the inhibition of monoamine oxidase by M & B 9302 (clorgyline)-11. Comparison of M & B 9302 inhibition with that of iproniazid. Biochem. Pharmacol. *18:* 1955–1959 (1969).

43 *Hall, D.W.R.; Logan, B.W., and Parsons, G.H.:* Further studies on the inhibition of monoamine oxidase by M & B 9302 (clorgyline)-1: Substrate specificity in various mammalian species. Biochem. Pharmacol. *18:* 1447–1454 (1969).

44 *Hanker, J.S.; Kusyk, C.J.; Bloom, F.E., and Pearse, A.G.E.:* The demonstration of dehydrogenases and monoamine oxidase by the formation of osmium blacks at the sites of Hatchett's Brown. Histochemie *33:* 205–230 (1973).

45 *Hardegg, W. und Heilbronn, E.:* Oxydation von Serotonin und Tyramin durch Rattenlebermitochondrien. Biochim. biophys. Acta *51:* 553–560 (1961).

46 *Hare, M.L.C.:* Tyramine oxidase. I. A new enzyme system in liver. Biochem. J. *22:* 968–979 (1928).

47 *Hartman, B.K.:* The discovery and isolation of a new monoamine oxidase from brain. Biol. Psychiat. *4:* 147–155 (1972).

48 *Hartman, B.K. and Udenfriend, S.:* The application of immunological techniques to the study of enzymes regulating catecholamines synthesis and degradation. Pharmacol. Rev. *24:* 311–330 (1972).

49 *Hartman, B.; Yasunobu, K.T., and Udenfriend, S.:* Immunological identity of the multiple forms of beef liver mitochondrial monoamine oxidase. Arch. Biochem. Biophys. *147:* 797–804 (1969).

50 *Hendley, E.D. and Snyder, S.H.:* Relationship between the action of monoamine oxidase inhibitors on the noradrenaline uptakes system and their anti-depressant officacy. Nature, Lond. *220:* 1330–1331 (1968).

51 *Holzbauer, M.; Bull, G.; Youdim, M.B.H.; Wooding, F.B.P., and Godden, U.:* Subcellular distribution of steroids in the adrenal gland. Nature New biol. *242:* 117–119 (1972).

52 *Holzbauer, M. and Youdim, M.B.H.:* Monoamine oxidase and oestrous cycle. Brit. Pharmacol. *48:* 600–608 (1973).

53 *Horita, A.:* The influence of pH on serotonin metabolism by rat tissue homogenates. Biochem. Pharmacol. *11:* 147–153 (1962).

54 *Houslay, M.D. and Tipton, K.F.:* The nature of the electrophoretically separable multiple forms of rat liver monoamine oxidase. Biochem. J. *135:* 173–186 (1973).

55 *Houslay, M.D. and Tipton, K.F.:* The reaction pathway of membrane-bound liver mitochondrial monoamine oxidase. Biochem. J. *135:* 735–750 (1973).

56 *Houslay, M.D. and Tipton, K.F.:* A kinetic evaluation of monoamine oxidase activity in rat liver mitochondrial outer membrane. Biochem. J. *139:* 645–652 (1974).

57 *Houslay, M.D.; Garrett, N.J., and Tipton, K.F.:* Mixed substrate experiments with human brain monoamine oxidase. Biochem. Pharmacol. *23:* 1937–1944 (1974).

58 *Iversen, L.L.:* Uptake and storage of noradrenaline in sympathetic nerves (Cambridge University Press, Cambridge 1967).

59 *Iversen, L.L.:* Catecholamine uptake processes. Brit. med. Bull. *29:* 130–135 (1973).

60 *Jarrott, B.:* Occurrence and properties of monoamine oxidase in adrenergic neurons. J. Neurochem. *18:* 7–16 (1971).

61 *Johnson, J.P.:* Some observations upon a new inhibitor of monoamine oxidase in brain tissue. Biochem. Pharmacol. *17:* 1285–1297 (1968).

62 *Kearney, E.B.; Salach, J.I.; Walker, W.H.; Seng, R.L.; Kenney, W.; Zeszotek, E., and Singer, T.P.:* The covalent bound flavin of hepatic monoamine oxidase. Isolation and sequence of a flavin peptide and evidence for binding of the 8α position. Europ. J. Biochem. *24:* 321–327 (1971).

63 *Klerman, G.L.:* Drug therapy of clinical depressions. Current status and implications for research on neuropharmacology of the affective disorders. J. Psychiat. Res. *9:* 253–270 (1972).

64 *Knoll, J. and Magyar, K.:* Some puzzling pharmacological effects of monoamine oxidase inhibitors. Adv. biochem. Psychopharmacol. *5:* 393–408 (1972).

65 *Knoll, J.; Ecseri, I.; Kelemen, K.; Nievel, J., and Knoll, B.:* Phenylisopropylmethyl-propinylamine (E-250). A new spectrum psychic energiser. Arch. int. pharmacol. Ther. *155:* 154–164 (1965).

66 *Kopin, I.J.:* Storage and metabolism of catecholamines. The role of monoamine oxidase. Pharmacol. Rev. *16:* 179–191 (1964).

67 *Kopin, I.J.:* Techniques for the study of alternate metabolic pathways of epinephrine metabolism in man. Science *131:* 1372–1374 (1960).

68 *Kopin, I.J. and Axelrod, J.:* The role of monoamine oxidase in the release and metabolism of norepinephrine. Ann. N.Y. Acad. Sci *107:* 848–855 (1963).

69 *Kroon, M.C. and Veldstra, H.:* Multiple forms of brain mitochondrial monoamine oxidase. FEBS Lett. *24:* 173–177 (1972).

70 *McCauley, R. and Racker, E.:* Separation of two monoamine oxidases from bovine brain. Molec. cell. Biochem. *1:* 73–81 (1973).

71 *Marley, E. and Blackwell, B.:* Inter-action of monoamine oxidase inhibitors, amines and foodstuffs. Adv. Pharmacol. *8:* 185–239 (1970).

72 *Meek, J.L. and Foldes, A.:* Sulfate conjugate in the brain; in *Usdin and Snyder* Frontiers in catecholamine research, pp. 167–172 (Pergamon Press, Oxford 1974).

73 *Murphy, D.L.:* Technical strategies for the study of catecholamines in man; in *Usdin and Snyder* Frontiers in catecholamine research (Pergamon Press, Oxford 1973).

74 *Murphy, D.L. and Donnelly, C.H.:* Monoamine oxidase in man. Enzyme characteristics in human platelets, plasma and other human tissues; in Neuropharmacology of monoamines and their regulatory enzymes, pp. 71–87 (Raven Press, New York 1974).

75 *Neff, N.H. and Goridis, C.:* Neuronal monoamine oxidase. Specific enzyme types and their rates of formation. Adv. Biochem. Psychopharmacol. *5:* 307–323 (1972).

76 *Neff, N.H. and Tozer, T.N.:* In *vivo* measurement of brain serotonin turnover. Adv. Pharmacol. *6A:* 97–109 (1968).

77   *Olivecrona, T. and Oreland, L.:* Reassociation of soluble monoamine oxidase with lipid-depleted mitochondria in the presence of phospholipid. Biochemistry *10:* 332–340 (1971).

78   *Oreland, L.:* Purification and properties of pig liver mitochondrial monoamine oxidase. Arch. Biochem. Biophys. *146:* 410–421 (1971).

79   *Oreland, L. and Ekstedt, B.:* Soluble and membrane-bound pig liver mitochondrial monoamine oxidase. Thermostability, tryptic digestibility and kinetic properties. Biochem. Pharmacol. *21:* 2479–2488 (1972).

80   *Pare, C.M.B.:* Potentiation of monoamine oxidase inhibitors by tryptophan. Lancet *ii:* 527–528 (1963).

81   *Pare, C.M.B.:* Clinical implications of monoamine oxidase inhibition. Adv. biochem. Psychopharmacol. *5:* 441–444 (1972).

82   *Pare, C.M.B.; Yeung, D.P.H.; Price, K., and Stacey, R.S.:* 5-Hydroxytryptamine, noradrenaline and dopamine in brain stem, hypothalamus and caudate nucleus of controls and of patients committing suicide by coal gas poisoning. Lancet *ii:* 133–135 (1969).

83   *Plelscher, A.; Gey, K.F., and Burkard, W.P.:* Inhibitors of monoamine oxidase and decarboxylase of aromatic amino acids; in: Handbook of experimental pharmacology, vol. 19, pp. 593–735 (Springer, Berlin 1966).

84   *Parvez, H. and Parvez, S.:* The regulation of monoamine oxidase activity by adrenal corticoid steroids. Acta endocrin. *73:* 509–517 (1973).

85   *Parvez, H. and Parvez, S.:* The effects of metopirone and adrenal ectomy on the regulation of the enzymes monoamine oxidase and catechol-*o*-methyl transferase in different brain regions. J. Neurochem. *20:* 1011–1020 (1973).

86   *Parvez, S.; Parvez, S.H., and Youdim, M.B.H.:* Variation in the activity of monoamine metabolizing enzyme in rat during pregnancy. Brit. J. Pharmacol. (in press).

87   *Ramey, E.R. and Goldstein, M.S.:* The adrenal cortex and the sympathetic nervous system. Physiol. Rev. *37:* 155–195 (1958).

88   *Robinson, D.S.; Davis, J.M.; Mies, A.; Colburn, R.W.; Davis, J.M.; Bourne, H.R.; Bunney, W.E.; Shaw, S.M., and Coppen, A.J.:* Ageing, monoamine and monoamine-oxidase levels. Lancet *i:* 290–291 (1972).

89   *Sandler, M. and Youdim, M.B.H.:* Multiple forms of monoamine oxidase. Functional significance. Pharmacol. Rev. *24:* 331–348 (1972).

90   *Sandler, M.; Collins, G.G.S., and Youdim, M.B.H.:* Inhibition pattern of monoamine oxidase isoenzymes. Clinical implications; in *Aldridge* Mechanism of toxicity (McMillan, London 1971).

91   *Sandler, M.; Youdim, M.B.H., and Hanington, E.:* A phenylethylamine oxidizing defect in migraine. Nature, Lond. *250:* 335–337 (1974).

92   *Schanberg, S.M.; Schildkraut, J.J., and Kopin, I.J.:* The effect of psychoactive drugs on norepinephrine-3H metabolism in brain. Biochem. Pharmacol. *16:* 393–399 (1967).

93   *Schayer, R.; Smiley, R.; Davis, K., and Kobayashi, Y.:* The metabolism of epinephrine containing isotopic carbon. J. biol. Chem. *198:* 545–551 (1952).

94   *Schayer, R.; Smiley, R.; Davis, K., and Kobayashi, Y.:* Role of monoamine oxidase in noradrenaline metabolism. Amer. J. Physiol. *182:* 285–291 (1955).

95   *Schnaitman, C.; Erwin, V.G., and Greenawalt, J.W.:* Submitochondrial localisation of monoamine oxidase. J. Cell. Biol. *34:* 719–735 (1967).

96   *Severina, I.S. and Gorkin, V.Z.:* On the nature of mitochondrial monoamine oxidase. Biokhimiya *28:* 896–902 (1963).

97   *Shore, P.A.; Mead, J.A.; Kuntzman, R.G.; Spector, S., and Brodie, B.B.:* On the physiological significance of monoamine oxidase in brain. Science *126:* 1063–1064 (1957).

98   *Singer, T.P.; Salach, J.I., and Youdim, M.B.H.:* The covalently bound flavin of brain monoamine oxidase (in preparation).

99   *Smith, I.; Kellow, A.H.; Mullen, P.E., and Hannington, E.:* Dietary migraine and tyramine metabolism. A possible inborn error of conjugation. Nature, Lond. *230:* 246–248 (1971).

100 *Southgate, J.:* Endometrial monoamine oxidase. The effect of sex steroids. Adv. biochem. Psychopharmacol. *5:* 263–270 (1972).

101 *Southgate, J.; Grant, E.C.G.; Pollard, W.; Pryse-Davies, J., and Sandler, M.:* Cyclic variation in endometrial monoamine oxidase. Correlation of histochemical and quantitative biochemical assays. Biochem. Pharmacol. *17:* 721–726 (1968).

102 *Spector, S.:* Monoamine oxidase in control of brain serotonin and norepinephrine content. Ann. N.Y. Acad. Sci. *107:* 856–864 (1963).

103 *Spector, S.; Tarver, J., and Berkowitz, B.:* Effects of drugs and physiological factors in the disposition of catecholamines in blood vessels. Pharmacol. Rev. *24:* 191–202 (1972).

104 *Spector, S.; Gordon, R.; Sjoerdsnid, A., and Udenfriend, S.:* End-product inhibition of tyrosine hydroxylase as a possible mechanism for regulation of norepinephrine synthesis. Molec. Pharmacol. *3:* 549–555 (1967).

105 *Spector, S.; Prockop, D.; Shore, P.A., and Brodie, B.B.:* Effect of iproniazid on brain levels of epinephrine and serotonin. Science *127:* 704–705 (1958).

106 *Squires, R.F.:* Additional evidence for the existence of several forms of mitochondrial monoamine oxidase in the mouse. Biochem. Pharmacol. *17:* 1401–1409 (1968).

107 *Symes, A.L.; Missala, K., and Sourkes, T.L.:* Iron- and riboflavin-dependent metabolism of a monoamine in the rat *in vivo.* Science *174:* 153–155 (1971).

108 *Symes, A.L.; Sourkes, T.L.; Youdim, M.B.H.; Gregoriadis, G., and Birnbaum, H.:* Decreased monoamine oxidase activity in liver of iron deficient rats. Canad. J. Biochem. *47:* 999–1003 (1969).

109 *Tabakoff, B.; Meyerson, L., and Alivisatos, S.G.A.:* Properties of monoamine oxidase in nerve endings from two bovine brain areas. Brain Res. *66:* 491–508 (1974).

110 *Tipton, K.F.:* The purification of pig brain mitochondrial monoamine oxidase. Europ. J. Biochem. *4:* 103–107 (1968).

111 *Tipton, K.F.:* Some properties of monoamine oxidase. Adv. biochem. Psychopharmacol. *5:* 11–24 (1972).

112 *Tipton, K.F.:* Biochemical aspects of monoamine oxidase. Brit. med. Bull. *29:* 116–119 (1973).

113 *Tipton, K.F.:* The adrenal gland; in *Blaschko and Smith* Handbook of physiology. 7. Endocrinology (The American Physiological Society, Washington 1975).

114 *Tipton, K.F.; Houslay, M.D., and Garrett, N.J.:* Allotopic properties of human brain monoamine oxidase. Nature New Biol. *246* 213–214 (1973).

115 *Tipton, K.F.; Youdim, M.B.H., and Spires, I.P.C.:* Beef adrenal medulla monoamine oxidase. Biochem. Pharmacol. *21:* 2197–2204 (1972).

116 *Tozer, T.N.; Neff, N.H., and Brodie, B.B.:* Application of steady-state kinetics to the synthesis rate and turnover time of serotonin in the brain of normal and reserpine treated rats. J. Pharmacol. exp. Ther. *153:* 177–182 (1966).

117 *Trendlelenburg, U.; Draskoćzy, P.R., and Graefe, K.H.:* The influence of intraneuronal monoamine oxidase on neuronal net uptake of noradrenaline and on sensitivity to noradrenaline. Adv. biochem. Psychopharmacol. *5:* 371–378 (1972).

118 *Usdin, E. and Snyder, S.H.:* Frontiers in catecholamine research (Pergamon Press, Oxford 1974).

118a *Weiner, N.:* The distribution of monoamine oxidase and succinic oxidase in brain. J. Neurochem. *6:* 79–86 (1960).

119 *Weiner, N. and Bjur, R.:* The role of intraneuronal monoamine oxidase in the regulation of norepinephrine synthesis. Adv. biochem. Psychopharmacol. *5:* 409–421 (1972).

120 *Walker, W.H.; Kearney, E.B.; Seng, R.L., and Singer, T.P.:* The covalently-bound flavin of hepatic monoamine oxidase. 2. Identification and properties of cysteinyl riboflavin. Europ. J. Biochem. *24:* 328–331 (1971).

121 *Wyatt, R.J.; Murphy, D.L.; Blemaker, R.; Cohen, S.; Donnelly, G.H., and Pollin, W.:* Reduced monoamine oxidase activity in platelets a possible genetic marker for vulnerability to schizophrenia. Science *179:* 916–917 (1973).

122 *Yang, H.Y.T. and Neff, N.H.:* β-phenylethylamine. A specific substrate for type B monoamine oxidase of brain. J. Pharmacol. exp. Ther. *187:* 365–371 (1973).

123 *Youdim, M.B.H.:* Multiple forms of monoamine oxidase and their properties. Adv. biochem. Psychopharmacol. *5:* 67–79 (1972).

124 *Youdim, M.B.H.:* Multiple forms of mitochondrial monoamine oxidase. Brit. med. Bull. *29.* 120–122 (1973).

125 *Youdim, M.B.H.:* Heterogeneity of rat brain and liver monoamine oxidase. Subcellular fractionation. Biochem. Soc. Trans. *1:* 1126–1127 (1973).

126 *Youdim, M.B.H.:* Monoamine deaminating system in mammalian tissues; in *Blaschko* MTP international review of science (Butterworths, London 1975).

127 *Youdim, M.B.H.:* Heterogeneity of rat brain mitochondrial monoamine oxidase. Adv. biochem. Psychopharmacol. *11:* 59–65 (1974).

128 *Youdim, M.B.H.:* Reporter's comments; in *Usdin and Snyder* Frontiers in catecholamine research, pp. 1184 (Pergamon Press, Oxford 1974).

129 *Youdim, M.B.H.:* Unpublished data.

130 *Youdim, M.B.H.:* Significance of selective inhibition of multiple forms of monoamine oxidase. J. Pharmacol., Paris *5* (1): 99 (1974).

130a *Youdim, M.B.H.:* The nature of brain monoamine oxidase. Proc. 9th Int. Congr. of Coll. Int. Neuropsychopharmacology (Excerpta Medica, Amsterdam 1975).

131 *Youdim, M.B.H. and Collins, G.G.S.:* The dissociation and reassociation of rat liver mitochondrial monoamine oxidase. Europ. J. Biochem. *18:* 73–78 (1971).

132 *Youdim, M.B.H. and Collins, G.G.S.:* Properties and physiological significance of multiple forms of mitochondrial monoamine oxidase (MAO); in *Markert* Isozymes (Academic Press, New York 1975).

133 *Youdim, M.B.H. and Collins, G.G.S.:* Monoamine oxidase inhibition and binding by phenelzinc. Biochem. Pharmacol. (in press).

134 *Youdim, M.B.H. and Hollman, B.:* The nature of brain monoamine oxidase inhibition by clorgyline (M & B 9302). (submitted for publication).

135 *Youdim, M.B.H. and Sourkes, T.L.:* The effect of heat, inhibitors and riboflavin deficiency on monoamine oxidase. Canad. J. Biochem. *43:* 1305–1318 (1965).

136 *Youdim, M.B.H. and Sourkes, T.L.:* Properties of purified soluble monoamine oxidase. Canad. J. Biochem. *44:* 1397–1400 (1966).

137 *Youdim, M.B.H.; Collins, G.G.S., and Sandler, M.:* Multiple forms of rat brain monoamine oxidase. Nature, Lond. *223:* 626–628 (1969).

138 *Youdim, M.B.H.; Holzbauer, M., and Woods, F.H.:* Neuropsychopharmacology of monoamines and their regulatory enzymes, pp. 11–28 (Raven Press, New York 1974).

139 *Youdim, M.B.H.; Bonham Carter, S.; Sandler, M.; Hannington, E., and Wilkinson, M.:* Conjugation defect in tyramine sensitive migraine. Nature, Lond. *230:* 127–129 (1971).

140 *Youdim, M.B.H.; Collins, G.G.S.; Sandler, M.; Bevan Jones, A.B.; Pare, C.M.B., and Nicholson, W.J.:* Human brain monoamine oxidase; multiple forms and selective inhibitors. Nature, Lond. *236:* 225–228 (1972).

141 *Youdim, M.B.H.; Woods, H.F.; Callender, S.; Mitchell, B., and Grahame-Smith, D.G.:* Human platelet monoamine oxidase activity in iron deficiency. Clin. Sci. Mol. Med. (in press).

142 *Zeller, E.A.:* Oxidation of amines; in *Sumner and Myrback* The enzyme chemistry and mechanism of action, vol. 2, pp. 536–558 (Academic Press, New York 1951).

Dr. *M.B.H. Youdim,* MRC Unit of Clinical Pharmacology, Radcliffe Infirmary, *Oxford OX2 6HE* (England)

Genetics and Psychopharmacology. Mod. Probl. Pharmacopsych., vol. 10, pp. 89–98,
ed. J. *Mendlewicz*, Brussels (Karger, Basel 1975)

A Genetic Study of Plasma Dopamine
β-Hydroxylase in Affective Disorder

Morton Levitt and Julien Mendlewicz

New York State Psychiatric Institute and Columbia University, New York, N.Y.

Introduction

Dopamine β-hydroxylase (DBH) catalyzes the terminal step in the biosynthesis of norepinephrine and is present in sympathetic neurons, brain and adrenal glands (*Kaufman and Friedman*, 1965). The enzyme is released on stimulation by a process termed 'exocytosis' in which particles or vesicles which contain norepinephrine and DBH migrate to the cell membrane and eject their contents to the exterior of the cell (*Viveros et al.*, 1968; *Gewirtz and Kopin*, 1970; *Axelrod*, 1972). It is believed that the DBH released in this way reaches the circulation. DBH activity can be measured in human serum or plasma (*Weinshilboum and Axelrod*, 1971 a; *Nagatsu and Udenfriend*, 1972). The plasma enzyme is identical in many ways with the enzyme found in tissues (*Weinshilboum et al.*, 1973 a).

DBH activity in humans varies over a wide range, however, in a given individual the enzyme activity is constant over long periods of time (*Weinshilboum and Axelrod*, 1971 a; *Goldstein et al.*, 1971; *Nagatsu and Udenfriend*, 1972; *Levitt et al.*, 1974). Plasma DBH activity increases for the first 5 years of life to adult levels with little subsequent increase (*Freedman et al.*, 1972; *Weinshilboum et al.*, 1973 b). *Horwitz et al.* (1973) reported that serum DBH activity was significantly higher in women as compared to men. In addition, these workers reported DBH activity to be lower in black than in white subjects.

Plasma enzyme activity is increased by exercise, postural changes and exposure to cold, which also increase sympathetic activity (*Vendsalu*, 1960; *von Eüler*, 1961; *Leduc*, 1961; *Mountcastle*, 1968; *Horwitz et al.*, 1973; *Wooten and Cardon*, 1973; *Frewin et al.*, 1973). However, the changes in DBH activity are small compared to the cardiovascular changes, and correlate poorly with other evidence of sympathetic function (*Horwitz et al.*, 1973).

Plasma or serum DBH activity has been studied in several diseases. In schizophrenics or affectively ill patients, both the range and mean of DBH activity is not different from the values obtained for a control population (*Wetterberg et al.*, 1972a; *Shopsin et al.*, 1972; *Dunner et al.*, 1973; *Levitt et al.*, in prep.). *Horwitz et al.* (1973) reported no significant difference between DBH values of hypertensive patients or control subjects; however, *Wetterberg et al.* (1972a) and *Schanberg et al.* (1973) reported higher levels or increased variability of DBH activity in hypertension. Reduced plasma levels of DBH activity were found in paraplegic and quadriplegic subjects (*Levitt et al.*, 1974).

Marked differences in plasma DBH activity have been reported in several genetic diseases. Patients with familial dysautonomia and Down's syndrome have low plasma DBH activity (*Weinshilboum and Axelrod*, 1971b; *Freedman et al.*, 1972; *Wetterberg et al.*, 1972b). Higher DBH activity was reported in autosomal dominant torsion dystonia and in Huntington's chorea (*Wooten et al.*, 1973; *Lieberman et al.*, 1972).

Recently, *Weinshilboum et al.* (1973b) demonstrated a high sibling-sibling correlation of serum DBH activity in normal children and adults. These workers also characterized a separate group of normals with very low serum DBH activity. *Ross et al.* (1973) found a high correlation coefficient for serum DBH activity in monozygotic twins and a slightly lower one for this activity in dizygotic twins. These observations suggest that plasma DBH activity is dependent on genetic factors. However, the mechanism which maintains and stabilizes the level of DBH activity in blood is poorly understood. Genetic control of release, stability or removal from the blood may regulate individual enzyme activity.

This report describes a comparative study of plasma DBH activity in monozygotic twins and same-sex siblings as well as in patients and relatives with affective illness. We had a 2-fold purpose in these studies, to further characterize the extent to which genetic factors control DBH activity and the exploration of the relationship between affective illness and plasma DBH activity.

Sample and Methods

The sample of twins (15 pairs, 8 females, 7 males, aged 29–65 years) was obtained by private referrals. Zygosity was established by physical traits and serological determinations (*Smith and Penrose*, 1955). The sample of siblings (12–80 years) was obtained from family studies of patients with both bipolar and unipolar depressive illness attending the Lithium Clinic at the New York State Psychiatric Institute.

The proband's diagnosis was made independently by 2 clinicians unaware of the family study data. The diagnostic criteria for both probands and their relatives are similar to those of *Leonhard et al.* (1962), *Angst and Perris* (1968) and *Winokur et al.* (1969). Bipolar illness was diagnosed in probands and relatives who had a history of manic behavior and of depressive episodes. Unipolar illness was diagnosed in individuals with depression only.

Blood samples were collected by vein puncture in heparinized tubes which were immediately placed on ice and centrifuged in the cold to separate the plasma. The samples were frozen at -80 °C until assayed. DBH activity was assayed by a modification of the spectrophotometric method described by *Nagatsu and Udenfriend* (1972). Duplicate 0.050-ml aliquots of each plasma sample were assayed. Cupric ions (1×10^{-6} M) were added to the incubation mixtures. The Dowex 50×8 H$^+$ colums were eluted with 3 ml of $3 N$ NH$_4$OH which was used in the subsequent determinations. Plasma DBH activity is expressed as μmol/min/l plasma. All correlations were calculated on the square roots of the plasma DBH activity as described by *Weinshilboum et al.* (1973b).

Results

Plasma DBH activity was measured in unipolar and bipolar patients. The study was conducted over a 10-month period and each patient was sampled 2–14 times (mean 4.5). The mean plasma DBH value for all patients was 55.7 ± 40.6 μmol/min/l plasma. This value compares with 53.3 ± 33.1 μmol/min/l plasma found in normal siblings of ill probands and 50.5 ± 37.9 μmol/min/l plasma found in 72 hypertensives. In our studies we found that individual plasma DBH values varied from undetectable levels (equal to background) to 180 μmol/min/l plasma. Both high and low values were found in all groups studied.

Plasma DBH activity in affectively ill patients is illustrated in table I. There is no significant difference between patients (male or female) diagnosed as unipolar or bipolar. These results are consistent with those of *Shopsin et al.* (1972) and *Wetterberg et al.* (1972a) who demonstrated that serum DBH activities of patients with affective illness are no different from controls. It is of interest that the plasma DBH activities found in 63 women (62.7 ± 41.1) were higher than those found in 51 men (47.2 ± 37.9). These results are consistant with those reported by *Horwitz et al.* (1973) who noted a sex difference.

The effect of lithium treatment on plasma DBH activity in affectively ill patients is shown in table II. Patients were treated with lithium carbonate in a double-blind study of affective episodes for 3 months to 3 years. The dose and

Table I. Plasma dopamine β-hydroxylase activity in patients with affective illness

Diagnosis	n	Males		n	Females	
		mean[1]	SD		mean[1]	SD
Unipolar	8	59.96	52.1	20	61.75	46.4
Bipolar	43	44.88	42.0	43	63.19	36.6

SD = standard deviation.
1 DBH activity, μmol/min/l plasma.

Table II. The effect of lithium on dopamine β-hydroxylase activity in patients with affective illness

	n	Mean[1]	SD	n	Mean[1]	SD
All patients	89	53.85	37.2	25	62.81	43.7
Unipolar	18	57.79	46.4	10	67.58	50.1
Bipolar	71	52.85	34.8	15	59.63	40.4

SD = standard deviation.
1 DBH activity μmol/min/l plasma.

Table III. Plasma dopamine β-hydroxylase (DBH) activity in same-sex siblings

Sibling	Sex	Dx (proband)	DBH activity[1]	
			proband	normal sibling
1	M	unipolar	34.8	61.8
2	F	bipolar	34.7	33.5
3	F	bipolar	8.5	10.4
4	M	bipolar	21.6	41.9
5	M	bipolar	21.8	17.6
6	M	unipolar	44.7	25.2
7	M	unipolar	65.8	85.7
8	F	unipolar	42.3	38.1
9	F	bipolar	123.0	133.3
10	F	bipolar	54.7	72.1
11	M	unipolar	25.4	40.3
12	F	unipolar	55.4	10.7
13	M	unipolar	69.5	80.2
14	F	bipolar	58.0	73.4
15	F	unipolar	99.7	104.4
16	M	unipolar	41.1	60.8
17	M	unipolar	43.8	14.1
18	M	unipolar	19.8	55.2
Mean DBH activity			48.01	53.31
SD			27.9	33.1

SD = standard deviation; Dx = diagnosis.
1 μmol/min/l plasma.

plasma concentrations of lithium were regularly monitored to obtain plasma levels of 0.8–1.3 mEq/l. There was no apparent relationship between those patients on lithium with respect to plasma DBH activity as compared to placebo patients. The values for plasma DBH activity in lithium-treated patients (unipolars and bipolars) are slightly lower than those in the placebo group but the difference is not significant. Furthermore, prospective studies of affectively ill patients failed to discern changes in plasma DBH activity during mood cycles (depression, mania and normothymia).

The relationship between affective illness and plasma DBH activity was further examined by comparing DBH values in pairs of same-sex siblings, one of whom was affectively ill and the other normal. Table III summarizes the results on 18 such pairs (10 males, 8 females). There is no difference in plasma DBH activity between well and ill siblings, regardless of the diagnosis of the ill sibling. It can be seen from table III that plasma DBH values in same-sex siblings are close to each other. Family studies have shown high sibling-sibling correlations of DBH activity (*Weinshilboum et al.,* 1973 a, b) and a high correlation in male monozygotic twins (*Ross et al.,* 1973). These observations suggest that plasma DBH activity is dependent on genetic factors. We have, therefore, studied plasma DBH activity in monozygotic twins and siblings in order to further characterize the extent to which genetic factors control plasma DBH activity.

The scatter plot of pairs of square-root values for 21 sets of siblings is illustrated in figure 1. The values for the two siblings who were closest in age

Table IV. Plasma dopamine β-hydroxylase (DBH) monozygotic twins

Twin pair	Sex	DBH activity[1]	
		proband	cotwin
1[2]	M	73.0	68.0
2	M	62.8	62.3
3	M	17.3	16.9
4[2]	M	36.2	33.6
5	F	103.5	92.1
6	F	60.9	62.3
7	F	28.9	29.9
8	F	101.1	99.2
9	F	101.2	93.8
10[2]	M	22.3	24.2
11	F	41.0	42.1
12[2]	M	37.5	38.1

1 μmol/min/l plasma.
2 Monozygotic twins discordant for affective illness.

were selected when a sibship consisted of more than 2 siblings. The resulting value of the product moment correlation coefficient, r = 0.33, is not significantly different from zero. However, in 5 pairs of sisters the correlation is r = 0.98 (p < 0.01). In 10 pairs of brothers it is r = 0.73 (p < 0.05). This value is equal to the one (r = 0.75) reported by *Ross et al.* (1973) for male dizygotic twins. In the brother-sister pairs, it is r = −0.42 (not significant). We find the correlation between a brother and a sister to be small compared to the correlation of same-sex siblings. *Weinshilboum et al.* (1973a) reported high sibling-sibling correlations of DBH activity regardless of sex.

The plasma DBH values for the 12 monozygotic twins (6 females and 6 males) are illustrated in table IV. There was no mean difference between males and females nor was there any association found with age. Four pairs of monozygotic twins discordant for affective illness were ascertained. The plasma DBH values are almost concordant in these twin pairs, indicating no influence of the affective disease on plasma DBH activity. When the square-root values of the plasma DBH activity of each twin pair were plotted the points clustered about a 45° line from the origin (fig. 2). This result indicates that the values for each twin pair are almost identical, the interclass correlation coefficient for all twin pairs combined is 0.99 (p < 0.001). This value is similar to the value (0.96) reported by *Ross et al.* (1973) for male monozygotic twins.

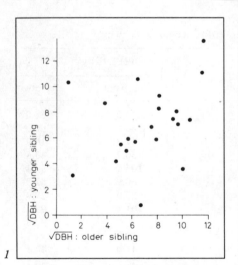
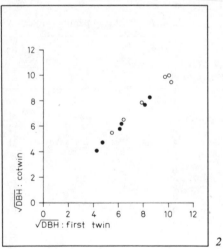

1   2

Fig. 1. Scatter plot of plasma dopamine β-hydroxylase (DBH) activity in 21 pairs of siblings. The square-root of DBH activity of each pair is illustrated.
Fig. 2. Scatter plot of plasma DBH activity in 12 pairs of monozygotic twins. The square-root of DBH activity is illustrated. ● = male pairs and ○ = female pairs.

The heritability estimate for plasma DBH activity was obtained by comparing the values for within twin pair variances with within same-sex sibling variances. Plasma DBH activity in males and females was found to have a heritability value greater than 0.90, which indicates a strong genetic influence.

Discussion

One of the more interesting findings in DBH activity studies is the narrow range of values shown by a given individual over time compared to the wide range of activity seen across different individuals (*Weinshilboum et al.*, 1973a; *Horwitz et al.* 1973). Small changes in plasma DBH activity have been reported after exercise, postural changes (tilt table), cold stress and during the menstrual cycle (*Wooten and Carden*, 1973; *Horwitz et al.*, 1973; *Frewin et al.*, 1973; *Levitt et al.*, 1974; *Lamprecht et al.*, 1974). Lithium carbonate used to treat mania or depression did not modify plasma DBH activity. Resting levels of plasma DBH activity in schizophrenics are not different from values obtained from control subjects (*Wetterberg et al.*, 1972; *Dunner et al.*, 1974).

A subgroup in the general population has been described to have low levels of plasma DBH activity; however, these individuals have normal sympathetic function (*Weinshilboum et al.*, 1973a, b; *Horwitz et al.*, 1973). Further, the entire spectrum of plasma DBH activity has been found among groups of hypertensives, manic-depressives and schizophrenics.

The small, and variable changes after stress and the wide range of values found in several disease states emphasize the difficulty of relating plasma DBH activity with the sympathetic system. These findings suggest that the value of plasma DBH activity as a sensitive monitor of the function of the sympathetic system is doubtful (*Horwitz et al.*, 1973; *Weinshilboum et al.*, 1973a, b).

Plasma DBH activity has been shown to differ from that of controls in several genetic diseases such as Down's syndrome (*Wetterberg et al.*, 1972b), autosomal dominant torsion dysotonia (*Wooten et al.*, 1973), Huntington's chorea (*Lieberman et al.*, 1972), and familial dysautonomia (*Weinshilboum and Axelrod*, 1971b). However, *Goldstein et al.* (1974) reported that concentrations of DBH in familial dysautonomia and torsion dystonia reflect genetic influences rather than pathology of the disease. *Weinshilboum et al.* (1973b) have demonstrated a highly significant correlation of DBH activity in pairs of sibs. Further, *Ross et al.* (1973) have shown a high concordance rate for DBH activity in male monozygotic twins and a lower, but significant, concordance rate in dizygotic twins. These results indicate that familial factors play an important role in controlling plasma or serum DBH activity. Further, environmental factors seem to have little influence on plasma DBH activity (*Horwitz et al.*, 1973a; *Wooten and Cardon*, 1973; *Frewin et al.*, 1973).

Our results for affectively ill probands and their first-degree relatives confirm and extend previous studies of plasma DBH activity in affective illness. The negative findings for plasma DBH activity in patients is strengthened by the equally negative findings in same-sex siblings and twins discordant for affective illness. Thus, the plasma DBH activity of unipolar or bipolar patients is not different from control values. The presence or absence of affective illness in paired siblings did not affect individual or group plasma DBH activity. Furthermore, 4 pairs of monozygotic twins discordant for affective illness were concordant for plasma DBH activity. The family and twin studies further confirm the lack of correlation between affective illness and plasma DBH activity and emphasize the genetic determination of the activity of this enzyme in plasma. Additional studies of plasma DBH activity in large families are in progress to characterize the mode of genetic transmission of this enzyme.

Summary

Plasma DBH activity was studied in patients with affective illness (unipolar or bipolar) and in their families. We found diagnosis, mood state or lithium treatment did not modify plasma DBH activity. In family studies we found same-sex siblings to show significant correlations for plasma DBH activity regardless of diagnosis. Monozygotic twins had almost identical DBH activities; 4 pairs of monozygotic twins discordant for affective illness were concordant for DBH activity. The heritability estimate for plasma DBH activity is greater than 0.90, indicating a strong genetic influence. These studies reveal that affective illness does not modify plasma DBH activity and that familial factors play an important role in controlling plasma DBH activity.

Acknowledgements

We wish to thank Ms. *E. Danielson* for her excellent technical assistance, and Dr. *W. Lawlor* and Dr. *J. Fleiss* for their statistical analysis of the data. We are greatful to Dr. *R.R. Fieve* and other members of the staff of the New York State Psychiatric Institute Lithium Clinic for their help. This study has been partly supported by Grant MH21586-03, from the National Institute of Mental Health.

References

Angst, J. und Perris, C.: Zur Nosologie endogener Depression. Vergleich der Ergebnisse der Untersuchungen. Arch. Psychiat. *210:* 373–386 (1968).

Axelrod, J.: Dopamine β Hydroxylase. Regulation of its synthesis and release from nerve terminals. Pharmacol. Rev. *24:* 233–243 (1972).

Dunner, D.L.; Cohn, C.K.; Weinshilboum, R.M., and Wyatt, R.J.: The activity of dopamine β hydroxylase and methionine activating enzyme in blood of schizophrenic patients. Biol. Psychiat. *6:* 215–220 (1973).

Endicott, J. and Spitzer, R.L.: Current and past psychopathology scales. Rationale, reliability and validity. Arch. gen. Psychiat. *27:* 678–687 (1972).

Eüler, C. Von: Physiology and pharmacology of temperature regulation. Pharmacol. Rev. *13:* 361–398 (1961).

Freedman, L.S.; Ohuchi, T.; Goldstein, M.; Axelrod, J.; Fish, I., and Dancis, J.: Changes in human serum dopamine-β-hydroxylase activity with age. Nature, Lond. *236:* 310, 311 (1972).

Frewin, D.B.; Downey, J.A., and Levitt, M.: The effect of heat, cold and exercise on dopamine β hydroxylase activity in man. Canad. J. Physiol. Pharmacol. *51:* 986–989 (1973).

Gewirtz, G.P. and Kopin, I.J.: Release of dopamine-β-hydroxylase with norepinephrine during cat splenic stimulation. Nature, Lond. *227:* 406, 407 (1970).

Goldstein, M.; Freedman, L.S., and Bonnay, M.: An assay for dopamine β hydroxylase activity in tissues and serum. Experientia *27:* 632, 633 (1971).

Goldstein, M.; Freedman, L.S.; Ebstein, R.P.; Park, D.H., and Kashimoto, T.: Human serum dopamine β hydroxylase. Relationship to sympathetic activity in physiological and pathological states. Psychopharm. Bull. *10:* 25 (1974).

Horwitz, D.R.; Alexander, R.W.; Lovenberg, W., and Keiser, H.: Human serum dopamine β hydroxylase. Circulat. Res. *32:* 594–599 (1973).

Kaufman, S. and Friedman, S.: Dopamine β hydroxylase. Pharmacol. Rev. *17:* 71–100 (1965).

Lamprecht, F.; Matta, R.J.; Little, B., and Zahn, T.D.: Plasma dopamine β hydroxylase (DBH) activity during the menstrual cycle. Psychosomat. Med. *36:* 304–310 (1974).

Leduc, J.: Catecholamine production and release in exposure and acclimation to cold. Acta physiol. scand. *53:* suppl. 183, pp. 22–46 (1961).

Leonhard, K.; Korff, I. und Shulz, H.: Die Temperamente in den Familien der monopolaren und bipolaren phasischen Psychosen. Psychiat. Neurol. *143:* 416–434 (1962).

Levitt, M.; Frewin, D.B.; Cayetano, C.; Co, C.C.; Luke, W., and Downey, J.A.: Plasma dopamine β hydroxylase activity in paraplegic and quadriplegic subjects. Austr. N.Z. J. Med. *4:* 48–52 (1974).

Levitt, M.; Dunner, D.L.; Mendlewicz, J.; Lawler, W.; Fleiss, J.L.; Frewin, D.B.; Stallone, F., and Fieve, R.R.: Plasma dopamine β hydroxylase activity in patients with affective disorder (in preparation).

Lieberman, A.N.; Freedman, L.S., and Goldstein, M.: Serum dopamine β hydroxylase activity in patients with Huntington's chorea and Parkinson's disease. Lancet *i:* 153, 154 (1972).

Mountcastle, V.B.: Medical physiology (Mosby, St. Louis 1968).

Nagatsu, T. and Udenfriend, S.: Photometric assay of dopamine-β-hydroxylase activity in human blood. Clin. Chem. *18:* 980–983 (1972).

Robins, E. and Guze, S.B.: Classification of affective disorders. The primary-secondary, the endogenous-reactive, and the neurotic-psychotic concepts; in *Williams, Katz and Shield* Recent advances in psychobiology of the depressive illness. DHEW Publication (HSM) 70–9053 (1972).

Ross, S.B.; Wetterberg, L., and Myrked, M.: Genetic control of plasma dopamine β hydroxylase. Life Sci. *12:* 529–532 (1973).

Schanberg, S.; Stone, R.; Kirschner, N.; Gunnels, J.C., and Robinson, R.R.: Plasma DBH. An aid in the study and diagnosis of hypertension. Pharmacologist *15:* 211 (1973).

Shopsin, B.; Freedman, L.S.; Goldstein, M., and Gershon, S.: Serum dopamine β hydroxylase (DBH) activity and affective states. Psychopharmacologia, Berl. *27:* 11–16 (1972).

Smith, S.M. and Penrose, L.S.: Monozygotic and dizygotic twin diagnosis. Ann. hum. Genet. *19:* 273–289 (1955).

Vendsalu, A.: Studies on adrenaline and noradrenaline in human plasma. Acta physiol. scand. *49:* suppl. 173, pp. 61–79 (1960).

Viveros, O.H.; Arqueros, L., and Kirshner, N.: Release of catecholamines and dopamine β hydroxylase from the adrenal medulla. Life Sci. *7:* 609–618 (1968).

Weinshilboum, R.M. and Axelrod, J.: Serum dopamine β hydroxylase activity. Circulat. Res. *28:* 307–315 (1971a).

Weinshilboum, R. and Axelrod, J.: Reduced plasma dopamine β hydroxylase in familial dysautonomia. N. Engl. J. Med. *285:* 938–942 (1971b).

Weinshilboum, R.M.; Raymond, F.A.; Elveback, L.R., and Weidman, W.H.: Dopamine β hydroxylase activity in serum; in *Usden and Snyder* Frontiers in catecholamine research (Pergamon Press, New York 1973a).

Weinshilboum, R.M.; Raymond, F.A., and Weidman, W.H.: Serum dopamine β hydroxylase activity. Sibling-sibling correlation. Science *181:* 943–945 (1973b).

Wetterberg, L.; Aberg, H.; Ross, S.B., and Fröden, O.: Plasma dopamine β hydroxylase activity in hypertension and various neuropsychiatric disorders. Scand. J. clin. Lab. Invest. *30:* 283–289 (1972a).

Wetterberg, L.; Gustavson, K.H.; Bäckström, M.; Ross, S.B., and Fröden, O.: Low dopamine β hydroxylase activity in Down's syndrome. Clin. Genet. *3:* 152, 153 (1972b).

Winokur, G.; Clayton, P.J., and Reich, T.: Manic depressive illness, p. 124 (Mosby, St. Louis 1969).

Wooten, G.F. and Cardon, P.V.: Plasma dopamine β hydroxylase activity. Arch. Neurol., Chicago *28:* 103–106 (1973).

Wooten, G.F.; Eldridge, R.; Axelrod, J., and Stern, R.S.: Elevated plasma dopamine β hydroxylase activity in autosomal dominant torsion dystonia. New Engl. J. Med. *288:* 284–287 (1973).

Dr. *M. Levitt* and Dr. *J. Mendlewicz,* New York State Psychiatric Institute, 722 W 168 St., *New York, NY 10032* (USA)

Genetics and Psychopharmacology. Mod. Probl. Pharmacopsych., vol. 10, pp. 99–132, ed. *J. Mendlewicz,* Brussels (Karger, Basel 1975)

Cytogenetic Effects of Psychoactive Drugs

Steven S. Matsuyama and Lissy F. Jarvik[1]

Veterans Administration Hospital (Brentwood), Los Angeles and Department of Psychiatry, University of California, Los Angeles, Calif.

Introduction

The consumption of pharmacological agents for pleasure and therapeutic purposes dates far back in history. Initially, these agents were limited to naturally occurring compounds. Today, chemically synthesized psychoactive agents have added greatly to the abundance and availability of drugs for the modification of human behavior.

Within our generation, pharmacotherapy has revolutionized the treatment of major mental disorders (psychoses). Pharmacological agents are also used by nonpsychotic persons to relieve tension, anxiety, and depression, and merely to enhance 'normal' experiences.

Possible deleterious effects of these agents on the hereditary material of man are of serious concern. Reports suggesting damage to chromosomes (breaks and/or other abnormalities) as a result of drug ingestion have been sufficiently disturbing to warrant testing for possible mutagenic, teratogenic, and/or carcinogenic effects. According to *Moorhead et al.* (1971), an elevated frequency of chromosomal aberrations may be considered a reliable indicator of the presence of genetic changes.

It has become increasingly clear that gross chromosomal aberrations are associated with various forms of malignant neoplasia. For example, patients who underwent arteriography with thorium dioxide, a radioactive substance containing isotopes of the thorium-232 decay series, show a high frequency of chromo-

---

1   The authors gratefully acknowledge the assistance of *Carole Morgan* and *Jane Granoff* in the preparation of the final manuscript.

some aberrations (*Fischer et al.,* 1967), and long-term follow-up studies have demonstrated a high frequency of carcinoma in these same individuals. An entirely different example is provided by persons afflicted with Down's syndrome (mongolism) who, since the advent of antibiotics, are able to survive intercurrent infections in early childhood and face a high risk of leukemia (*Miller,* 1970). It is believed that the extra chromosomal material in these patients (chromosome 21) may be responsible for the tendency to malignant neoplasia. Subjects with Bloom's syndrome and Fanconi's anemia constitute other groups where an elevated frequency of chromosome aberrations is associated with a high incidence of acute leukemia (*German,* 1969; *Swift and Hirschhorn,* 1966; *Hirschhorn and Bloch-Shtacher,* 1970; *Swift,* 1971). There is also the aberration known as the Philadelphia chromosome which is considered specific for chronic myelogenous leukemia, for it is observed only in this condition (*de Grouchy,* 1967; *Knudson et al.,* 1973). Whether chromosome abnormalities are the cause or the result of malignant tranformations, or both are caused by a common factor, is important, but not as important as the fact that an altered genome can provide cells with unlimited growth potential, and thus allow for the progression of tumors.

Presently, cytogenetic analysis constitutes the best available procedure for the *in vivo* testing of effects of drugs or other environmental agents on the genetic material of man. Human cytogenetics is a relatively new field. It was only in 1956 that the full chromosomal complement of man was determined (*Tjio and Levan,* 1956). It was even later that *Moorhead et al.* (1960) introduced human peripheral leukocyte cultures which, with modifications, constitute the technique most frequently used throughout the world for both *in vivo* and *in vitro* testing of drug effects on the human genome.

Two other cell types, bone marrow cells and fibroblasts, are also used in assessing the effects of drugs. Direct examination of bone marrow reflects *in vivo* effects, while fibroblast cultures permit long-term *in vitro* testing. However, in both cases, the procurement of cells for analysis requires special procedures (bone marrow aspiration or skin biopsy) in contrast to blood samples for leukocyte cultures which can be readily obtained from subjects, and repeat determinations easily made with little risk and discomfort to the individual. Therefore, leukocyte cultures have generally been preferred.

Although the human peripheral leukocyte culture technique is relatively simple, leukocytes are somatic cells and do not provide information on gonadal cells which are of primary genetic importance. Yet, *any* evidence of genetic damage may be indicative of similar damage in gonadal cells, and a drug causing such damage may, therefore, be considered potentially deleterious to future generations as well as a health risk to the individual himself. The inability of cytogenetic analysis to detect point mutations that may be induced by various compounds suggests an underestimate rather than an overestimate of the total mutagenic effect. In this regard, *Nichols* (1973) believes that chromosomal damage is a good indicator of mutagenesis, stating that there is a 'high correlation between the ability of an agent to produce gene mutations and its ability to produce chromosome breakage'.

Inherent in cytogenetic testing is the ability to detect, under the microscope, visible morphological changes in the metaphase chromosomes. The recent discovery of techniques which make possible the identification of each chromosome by its characteristic banding pattern has brought cytogenetic analysis to new heights. (For a review of various techniques, see *Miller et al.,* 1973.) With these techniques, chromosome rearrangements, as a result of chromosome breaks caused by drug ingestion, are easily discernible, if present.

It is uncertain what importance should be attached to increased chromosome breaks detected in leukocyte cultures. Cells with breaks may be eliminated, or breaks may be repaired by simple rejoining. In either case, no detrimental effect is necessarily expected. It is only if cells with damaged chromosomes are sequestered and later come to expression as malignant neoplasia, or if damaged gonadal cells, upon fertilization, give rise to offspring with congenital anomalies that chromosome breaks become important. Therefore, cytogenetic monitoring is recommended so that potentially deleterious effects of drugs may be detected early.

With the above relationships in mind, a survey of the literature was undertaken and the following questions were considered: (1) What is available in the literature on the cytogenetic effects of psychoactive drugs? (2) Which drugs, if any, are capable of causing chromosome damage *in vivo* and/or *in vitro?* (3) For which drugs examined for mutagenicity is there evidence for or against teratogenicity?

It was noted, as in a previous extensive survey dating to 1970 (*Moorhead et al.,* 1971), that much of the information available was only assertion of fact without accompanying data, mere statement of opinion, editorial commenting, or interpretation of other investigators' findings, and expansion of earlier publications by the same investigators. Therefore, care was taken in determining the number of studies and subjects actually contributing to the data on cytogenetic effects of drugs lest they be overestimated by being counted more than once.

The following review of the cytogenetic literature on the more commonly used or abused psychoactive agents includes hallucinogens (LSD and marijuana); opiates (heroin, morphine, and methadone); antipsychotic drugs (phenothiazines: chlorpromazine, fluphenazine, perphenazine, and thioridazine; and lithium); antianxiety drugs (meprobamate, chlordiazepoxide, and diazepam); antidepressants (imipramine), and anticonvulsants.

It is hoped that by gathering the relevant literature, an accurate impression will be gained of the present knowledge, and the gaps in knowledge, about the effects of these drugs on the hereditary material of man, and the potential danger to present 'users' and to future generations.

Table I. Comparison of chromosome analyses in LSD 'users' and controls

Author	Year	LSD 'users'				
		subjects	age range years	cells analyzed	mean % breaks	range
Cohen et al.	1967a	18	19–52	4,282	13.2	5.3–25.1
Loughman et al.	1967	8	–	697	0.0	0
Abbo et al.	1968	2	19–20	60	10.0	6.7–13.3
Cohen et al.	1968	14	17–32	1,833	7.0	1.0–14
Egozcue et al.	1968	46[2]	17–43	9,140	18.8	8–45
Hulten et al.	1968	2	23–24	200	3.0	1.0–5.0
Jarvik et al.	1968	1	19	101	1.0	–
Sparkes et al.	1968	4	19–24	937	2.2	0.9–3.4
Judd et al.	1969	9	21–52	315	0.3	0–2.9
		8[4]	26–44	280	1.8	0–11.4
Nielsen et al.	1969	10	19.8 ± 3.0	635	2.5	–
Valenti	1969	10	15–25	894	2.0	0–5.8
Dorrance et al.	1970	14	17–27	1,284	0.8	0–2.0
Hsu et al.	1970	2	22–26	66	3.0	2.8–3.3
Stenchever and Jarvis	1970	12	18–31	2,525	1.3[5]	0–3.8
Dishotsky et al.	1971	14	–	1,412	0.4	–
Gilmour et al.	1971	8	–	400	1.2[5]	–

1 Two subjects with viral infections eliminated (14 and 31 % breaks).
2 Includes subjects reported by *Irwin and Egozcue* (1967).
3 Less two subjects with possible other drug use (18.5 and 24 % breaks).
4 Former users.
5 Percent cells with aberrations.

LSD

By far the most intensively studied agents are the hallucinogens, in particular LSD. The initial report on LSD was made by *Cohen et al.* (1967b) and showed that LSD was capable of causing extensive chromosome damage when added *in vitro*, and also *in vivo* as judged by the findings in one male schizophrenic following its use in treatment. This alarmed the public and medical community who had only recently weathered the thalidomide incident, and led to an intensive investigation of the effects of LSD on chromosomes. Yet, after 7 years of research and numerous publications there still remains the controversy as to the potential of LSD to cause chromosome damage. In an attempt to examine this controversy anew, the data in the various reports have been arranged into four groups: (1) LSD 'users' (i.e. users of illicit or street-obtained LSD with its attendant impurities and imprecise dosage); (2) medically treated

Table I (continued)

Author	Year	Controls				
		subjects	age range years	cells analyzed	mean % breaks	range
Cohen et al.	1967a	12[1]	22–55	2,674	3.8	2.0–5.5
Loughman et al.	1967	19	–	673	0.4	–
Abbo et al.	1968	32	24–59	1,022	3.5	0–?
Cohen et al.	1968	9	20–35	1,203	1.2	0–2.0
Egozcue et al.	1968	14	–	2,800	9.0	6.0–16.5
Hulten et al.	1968	5	0.5–38	250	2.4	0–6.0
Jarvik et al.	1968	11[3]	22–61	720	4.7	0–9.0
Sparkes et al.	1968	4	21–50	950	1.6	0.8–2.6
Judd et al.	1969	8	17–48	280	0.7	0–5.7
Nielsen et al.	1969	30	31.4 ± 9	1,030	0.2	–
Dorrance et al.	1970	10	18–44	1,018	0.8	0–2.0
Stenchever and Jarvis	1970	8	17–45	1,620	1.1	0–3.0
Dishotsky et al.	1971	8	–	805	0.6	–
Gilmour et al.	1971	16	–	771	0.5[5]	–

LSD subjects; (3) cytogenetic findings in infants exposed *in utero* to LSD (illicit and pure), and (4) *in vitro* studies. Finally, animal studies will be briefly reviewed.

Human Studies

LSD users. There are at least 16 studies of LSD users published in the literature. However, the lack of an adequate number of subjects in many of the studies (i.e. reports on only one or two subjects), makes it impossible to assign an equal weight to all studies for comparative purposes. Therefore, we have restricted our review to the ten studies reporting eight or more subjects, but for completeness have listed all studies in table I. Although *Valenti* (1969) reported on ten subjects, a control group was not available for comparison. Of the ten studies with a sample size of eight or more, five showed an increased frequency of breaks or aberrant cells (*Cohen et al.*, 1967a, 1968; *Egozcue et al.*, 1968;

Table II. Comparison of chromosome analyses in subjects medically treated with LSD and controls

Author	Year	Treated with LSD				
		subjects	age range years	cells analyzed	mean % breaks	range
Cohen et al.	1967b	1[1]	51	200	12.0	–
Abbo et al.	1968	5	24–57	266	8.3	3.3–13.3
Hungerford et al.[2]	1968	4[3,5]	–	1,375	3.9	1.0–7.0
		4[4,5]	–	350	1.1	0–6.0
Nielsen et al.	1968	5	29–48	358	1.7	0–6.9
Sparkes et al.	1968	4	28–45	914	1.5	0.4–2.5
Nielsen et al.	1969	9	36.1 ± 7.2	603	4.3	–
Siva Sankar et al.[7]	1969	15	7–15	1,500	0.8	0–2.0
		7[8]	7–15	700	1.0	0–3.0
Tjio et al.[9]	1969	11[10]	21–50	2,347	9.3	2.0–43.9
		21[11]	20–56	4,387	4.2	1.5–14.2
		5	23–35	–	3.2	1.0–5.7
		8	–	1,646	2.8	2.0–3.8
Corey et al.	1970	10[12]	–	1,000	4.9	2.0–8.0
		5	–	500	7.8	6.0–12.0
		6[13]	–	594	6.4	2.0–11.0
Warren et al.	1970	2	36–37	–	NSI[14]	–
Dishotsky et al.	1971	5	–	500	0.4	–
Fernandez et al.	1973	32	18–48	4,099	0.6	0–3.2
Jarvik et al.	1974	2[4]	24–45	800	1.4	0–3.0
		6[3]	24–45	1,650	2.2	0–4.0

1 Also used other drugs.
2 Intravenous administration.
3 During LSD bloods combined.
4 Combined follow-up bloods.
5 Chlorpromazine, 100 mg tablet prior to LSD.
6 Additional controls.
7 Includes *Bender and Siva Sankar* (1968).

Nielsen et al., 1969; *Gilmour et al.*, 1971), while five did not (*Loughman et al.*, 1967; *Judd et al.*, 1969; *Dorrance et al.*, 1970; *Stenchever and Jarvis*, 1970; *Dishotsky et al.*, 1971). In all of the above reports, no relationship was seen between chromosome damage and dosage, number of doses, duration of use, total amount used, and the interval from the last dose to chromosome analysis. The necessity to rely on the subjects' ability to recall their use patterns makes this information suspect, and is estimated rather than hard data. Furthermore, it is difficult to assess the true dosage in illicitly obtained LSD. Indeed, *Krippner*

Table II (continued)

Author	Year	Controls				
		subjects	age range years	cells analyzed	mean % breaks	range
Cohen et al.	1967b	–	–	–	3.7	–
Abbo et al.	1968	32	24–59	1,022	3.5	0–?
Hungerford et al.[2]	1968	3	–	600	1.0	1.0–7.0
		3[6]	–	900	1.2	0–3
Nielsen et al.	1968	40	17–59	1,312	0.4	–
Sparkes et al.	1968	4	21–50	950	1.6	0.8–2.6
Nielsen et al.	1969	30	31.4 ± 9	1,030	0.2	–
Siva Sankar et al.[7]	1969	25	7–15	2,500	0.7	–
		7	20–43	700	0.6	–
Tjio et al.[9]	1969	11	21–50	2,294	4.1	2.0–9.5
		21	20–56	4,404	4.4	1.5–19.4
		5	–	–	2.8	1.5–3.8
		2[6]	30–38	–	2.6	1.5–4.8
Corey et al.	1970	10	–	1,000	5.7	1.0–9.0
		13	–	1,300	7.0	2.0–17.0
		–	–	–	–	–
Warren et al.	1970	–	–	–	–	–
Dishotsky et al.	1971	8	–	805	0.6	–
Fernandez et al.	1973	32	age matched ± 5 years	4,271	0.4	0–1.6
Jarvik et al.	1974	2	24–45	200	2.5	2.0–3.0

8 UML (4.54 mg/day) also administered together with LSD. One patient with 9 % breaks not included.
9 Data are percent abnormal cells and not percent breaks.
10 Low dose (50 µg).
11 High dose (250–450 µg).
12 Pre- and post-bloods – subject serves as own control.
13 Also received mescaline.
14 No significant increase over controls.

(1970), on analyzing 12 tablets obtained from various sources and reportedly sold as containing 250 µg LSD, found one tablet without any LSD, and only two with more than 150 µg. Most contained less than 26 µg, and many had more STP (DOM) than LSD. Since it is most likely that many impurities are contained in illicitly obtained tablets, and since there have been frequent reports of the use of other drugs along with LSD, one concludes that drug users in general, and not specifically LSD users, show an elevated rate of chromosome breaks. In addition, personal hygiene, diet, general living conditions and exposure to infection differ between controls and users, and may be directly responsible for increased chromosome damage found in LSD users. *Cohen et al.* (1967a) for example, eliminated two subjects with viral infections from their control population who showed 14 and 31 % breaks. The frequency of structural abnormalities roughly paralleled that of breaks, and structural abnormalities were seen in controls as well as drug users.

In the only study of human meiotic chromosomes, *Hulten et al.* (1968) could not demonstrate an elevated frequency of chromosomal abnormalities in the testicular material of one man.

Medically administered LSD. There are 13 reports of chromosome analyses on individuals administered LSD under medical supervision (table II). These studies are of two types. One type compares LSD-treated individuals to a separate control group. In the second type, subjects are studied before, during, and after treatment, thus serving as their own control. For purposes of comparison, we have focused our attention on those studies reporting five or more subjects. Six studies are of the first type, and three detected a statistically significant increase in chromosome breaks (*Abbo et al.,* 1968; *Nielsen et al.,* 1968, 1969). However, these are based on only 19 subjects, 14 of them from one laboratory. *Nielsen* also reported elevated frequencies of breaks in illicit users of LSD.

There are four reports of the second type which approach a scientifically sound experimental design to assess the chromosome damaging potential of LSD (*Hungerford et al.,* 1968; *Tjio et al.,* 1969; *Corey et al.,* 1970; *Jarvik et al.,* 1974). Pure LSD of known dosages was administered to subjects with chromosome examinations at specified intervals prior to, during, and following treatment. *Hungerford et al.* (1968) reported on three subjects for whom blood samples for chromosome analyses were taken 1 h before, during the course of treatment (three treatments at 1–2 week intervals), and 1–6 months following the last LSD administration. For a fourth subject, no predrug culture was available for analysis. In this study, LSD was administered intravenously at doses of 187–200 µg/treatment. Three control subjects matched for age and sex were also studied with three chromosome examinations for each at 1 week intervals. The mean percent breaks in these controls was 1.2 % (range of 0–3 %).

In LSD-treated individuals, the pretreatment mean was 1.0 %, during LSD treatment 3.9 %, and 1.1 % in follow-up examinations. Hence, the data suggest a transient increase in breaks with a return to predrug levels 1–6 months following termination of treatment. A number of structural abnormalities were recorded and these were seen only after LSD treatment had started, none having been observed in pretreatment cultures, or in control subjects.

In the second study, *Tjio et al.* (1969) reported on 32 subjects given a single dose of LSD orally (11 given 50 µg and 21 given 250–450 µg). 200 cells were analyzed for each culture. No dose response relationship was seen. Of the eleven low dose subjects, pre- and postdrug values (mean % aberrant cells) were 4.1 and 9.3 % while in the high dose group the values were 4.4 and 4.2 %, respectively. The combined frequency of aberrant cells for both groups was 4.3 % pre-LSD and 5.9 % post-LSD. Although there was a slight increase in aberrant cells, this was not statistically significant. 31 of the 32 subjects were also exposed to other drugs during their hospitalization. Seven of them were on drugs at the time pre-LSD blood was drawn, but none showed an unusually high frequency of aberrations. Four had documented viral infections and only one had an extremely high aberration rate (43.9 %). An additional five LSD users, who were given pure LSD in known dosages as part of an NIH study, also failed to show a statistically significant increase in breaks (2.8 vs. 3.2 %, pre- and postdrug cultures). In addition, eight individuals studied after LSD use showed no significant increase in comparison to controls. Structural abnormalities were recorded in both pre- and post-LSD cultures. Data were also presented on two normal drug-free subjects which show the day-to-day variations in the frequency of chromosomal abnormalities in the same individual. In one subject with nine successive determinations the range was from 1.48 to 3.38 %, and in the second subject with eight cultures, from 1.96 to 4.76 %. In support of the findings by *Tjio et al.* (1969), *Corey et al.* (1970) reported no increase in breaks in ten subjects on whom blood samples were drawn immediately before and 24 h after a single LSD administration. The frequency of structural abnormalities was significantly reduced in post-LSD cultures and they were only found in those individuals who manifested them initially.

In the final report (*Jarvik et al.,* 1974), two subjects for whom pre- and post-LSD values were available showed, if anything, a reduction in mean break frequency after receiving LSD, dextroamphetamine or placebo. Six additional subjects with no pre-LSD values also failed to show an increase in breaks during LSD treatment.

Therefore, in all prospective studies carried out (4), no definitive evidence has been presented that LSD damages lymphocyte chromosomes *in vivo. Hungerford et al.* (1968) did report a transient increase but in follow-up cultures all returned to pre-LSD values.

In utero exposure. *Idanpaan-Heikkila and Schoolar* (1969), using radioactive LSD, presented evidence that LSD crosses the placenta in mice, thereby exposing the fetus. Nine reports are available on chromosome analyses on infants exposed to LSD *in utero* (table III). Doses *in utero* ranged from none (*Cohen et al.,* 1968, reports on four infants whose mothers took LSD only prior to conception) to 30 or more (*Aase et al.,* 1970). Of the 73 infants studied, one had a limb anomaly and one presented an aberrant karyotype (*Hsu et al.,* 1970). Again, only *Cohen et al.* (1968) and *Egozcue et al.* (1968) reported an elevated rate of chromosome damage. It is difficult to assess the action of LSD since most

Table III. Chromosome examinations in infants exposed to LSD *in utero*

Author	Year	Subjects	Age range	Cells analyzed	Mean % breaks	Range	*In utero* doses
Abbo et al.	1968	1[1]	3 days	60	3.3	–	twice during 1st trimester
Cohen et al.[2]	1968	9	0.17–5.5 years	1,625	8.6	0–19	1–30
		4	0.5–4.0 years	568	4.0	2.0–8.7	LSD prior to conception only
		6	0.3–2.0 years	800	1.2	0–2.4	controls
Egozcue et al.	1968	4	1–18 months	800	21.5	9.5–28	1–6
Hulten et al.	1968	1	5 weeks	100	13	–	1,600 mg total exposure *in utero*
			8 months	100	4	–	
Aase et al.	1970	10	within 48 h of birth	500	no evidence of damage	–	1–30?
Hsu et al.	1970	1	1.5 years	40[3]	0	–	LSD prior to conception only
Stenchever and Jarvis	1970	1	8 months	28	0	–	twice only during 2nd trimester
Warren et al.	1970	1	birth to 3 months	–	0	–	exposure during 1st 4 months
Dumars	1971	41		2,050	1.5	–	?
		20	–	1,000	1.0	–	controls

1 Born with limb anomaly.
2 Includes 4 subjects from *Cohen et al.* (1967 a).
3 D-trisomy with congenital abnormalities.

mothers also took other drugs during their pregnancies, marijuana being one of the most prominent.

The potential teratogenic effect of LSD is far from clear. A survey of the literature led to reports on 244 children born to LSD users (*Aase et al.*, 1970; *Abbo et al.*, 1968; Anonymous, 1967; *Assemany et al.*, 1970; *Carakushansky et al.*, 1969; *Cohen et al.*, 1967a, 1968; *Dumars*, 1971; *Eller and Morton*, 1970; *Gelhrter*, 1970; *Hecht et al.*, 1968; *Hsu et al.*, 1970; *Hulten et al.*, 1968; *Jacobsen and Berlin*, 1972; *McGlothlin et al.*, 1970; *Sato and Pergament*, 1968; *Warren et al.*, 1970; *Zellweger et al.*, 1967). Of these, 213 were normal, seven were identified as cases of familial defects, and 24 (9.8 %) manifested congenital abnormalities. Six of the 24 were cases of limb deficiencies and further monitoring is warranted. However, most parents also used marijuana extensively making it difficult to indict LSD specifically. Extra care must be exercised in evaluating the literature since an inherent sample bias is present (i.e., malformed fetuses born to LSD users are reported more frequently than are normal infants born to LSD users, and more frequently than malformed infants born to normal drug-free individuals).

In vitro. There are eight reports of chromosome analyses following *in vitro* addition of LSD to lymphocyte cultures (table IV). Five reported an increase in breaks while three did not. All of the latter include only one or two subjects. Individual differences in susceptibility to chromosome breaks may constitute an important variable so far not sufficiently explored. In none of the positive studies was a dose response curve generated. The lowest dose tested was capable of producing the maximum damage possibly because low enough doses have not been tested. With one exception, the lowest dose tested, 0.001 μg/ml, was ten times higher than is calculated to be present in blood following ingestion of 100 μg LSD by a 70-kg man, and in that one exception, *Kato and Jarvik* (1969) did not find an increase in the frequency of breaks at a concentration of 0.0001 μg/ml. In general, it does appear that *in vitro* addition of LSD results in chromosome damage. However, care must be exercised in attempting to extrapolate *in vitro* results to *in vivo* findings. Drugs added to cells in culture are not subject to the body's metabolism and are readily available to the cells. Hence, they may act in a different manner than *in vivo*. Agents which exert a harmful effect *in vitro* may be detoxified and rendered harmless when consumed by the intact organism. And there is no reason to believe that the opposite situation may not also occur.

Animal Studies

The effects of LSD on the chromosomes of mice, rats, kangaroo rats, monkeys, and *Drosophila* have been reported.

Cohen and Mukherjee (1968), *Skakkebaek et al.* (1968) and *Skakkebaek*

Table IV. Chromosome analyses following *in vitro* addition of LSD. Survey of eight studies

Author	Year	No LSD added				
		subjects	age range years	cells analyzed	mean % breaks	range
Cohen et al.[1]	1967a	6	–	1,680	3.9	–
Jarvik et al.	1968	8	22–61	–	5.2	0–9.0
Mackenzie and Stone	1968	5	–	187	4.3[3]	–
Genest	1969	1	–	26	15	–
Kato and Jarvik	1969	2	–	100	5.0	–
Sturelid and Kihlman	1969	2	–	329	0.0	0
Corey et al.	1970	10	–	1,000	4.7	0–15.1
Jarvik et al.	1974	8	25–45	1,550	2.0	0.8–3.0

1 Includes *Cohen et al.* (1967b).
2 Two subjects showed no response.
3 Percent damaged cells.

and Beatty (1970) examined meiotic chromosomes in mice following LSD administration and detected a marked increase in abnormalities. *Cohen and Mukherjee* (1968) also studied bone marrow cells of LSD-treated mice and found a significant increase in structural aberrations, and a more than three-fold increase in breaks as compared to controls. However, *Egozcue and Irwin* (1969) and *Jagiello and Polani* (1969) could not replicate these observations, both reporting negative results.

All three studies available for rats had negative results. *Goetz et al.* (1972) studied meiotic chromosomes in male rats and found no increase in breaks with LSD. LSD administered orally (*Sato et al.,* 1971) and intraperitoneally (*Emerit et al.,* 1972) to pregnant rats produced no chromosome damage either in the mothers' bone marrow cells or in their embryos.

Bick (1970) found increased chromosome damage in leukocyte cultures of kangaroo rats following *in vitro* addition of LSD.

In monkeys *(Macaca mulatta),* the chromosomal effects of LSD were assessed *in vitro* and *in vivo. Egozcue and Irwin* (1969) reported a statistically significant increase in chromosome damage following *in vitro* treatment of leukocyte cultures. However, examinations of meiotic chromosomes prior to and following acute or chronic treatment showed no significant increase. By contrast, blood cultures of monkeys treated *in vivo* showed a significant increase in breaks including structural abnormalities.

Table IV (continued)

LSD added					LSD information	
subjects	age range years	cells analyzed	mean % breaks	range	dosages µg/ml	duration of exposure, h
6	–	7,735	13.0	7.7–17.5	10, 1, 0.1, 0.01, 0.001	4, 24, 48
8[2]	22–61	498	10.2	0.0–15.0	0.01	4
5	–	453	7.7[3]	7.2–8.3	0.1, 0.01	48
1	–	64	12.5	7.1–20.8	10, 1.0, 0.1	24
2	–	600	5.0	2.0–12.0	1, 0.01, 0.0001	4, 24
2	–	372	0.3	0–0.5	10	24, 48
10	–	1,000	9.4	4.0–18.7	1	24
8	25–45	4,320	3.4	1.7–6.0	0.1, 0.01, 0.001	4

Kato et al. (1970) examined leukocyte chromosomes of four pregnant Rhesus macaques following LSD administration. Two additional monkeys served as controls. The two monkeys receiving the highest doses of LSD showed a transient increase in breaks paralleling the results of *Hungerford et al.* (1968) in humans. Monkeys receiving low doses did not exhibit chromosome damage. Further, no structural abnormalities were found in postdrug cultures.

The two control monkeys gave birth to normal offspring. However, of the four LSD-treated monkeys, two pregnancies ended in stillbirths and one offspring died of pneumonia 1 month after birth. The only survivor of an LSD-treated mother showed no increase in chromosome damage. The potential meaning of this high incidence of mortality in offspring of LSD-treated mothers is uncertain since these animals were en route from Asia during their pregnancy; further investigation is warranted.

Three studies have been reported on the potential mutagenic and chromosome damaging effects of LSD in *Drosophila. Grace et al.* (1968) reported no increase in mutations and/or translocations as a result of intra-abdominal injection of LSD into *Drosophila* males. *Tobin and Tobin* (1969) likewise found no increase in lethals in the progeny of males who were injected during the meiotic and postmeiotic stages of spermatogenesis, or from larval feeding experiments. Finally, *Browning* (1968) reported a marked induction of recessive lethals following intraperitoneal injection of extremely high dosages of LSD.

Table V. Reports of chromosome analyses in persons exposed to psychiatric drugs and controls

Author	Year	Users				
		subjects	age range years	cells analyzed	mean % breaks	range
Marijuana						
Dorrance et al.	1970	9	19–27	816	0.9	0–2.7
Gilmour et al.	1971	13[1]	–	650	0.8[3]	–
		11[2]	–	550	2.2[3]	–
Rubin et al.	1973	30[4]	–	–	2.4[5]	–
Stenchever et al.	1974	49[4]	17–34	4,900	3.4[3]	0–8.0
Opiates						
Gilmour et al.	1971	11	–	650	2.2[3]	–
Falek et al.	1972	16[6]	21–58	861	0.2	–
		16[7]	21–58	1,173	2.6	–
Falek and McFadden	1973	13	21–29	1,456	4.5[8]	0–10.7
Abrams and Liao	1974	16[10]	–	1,600	11.4	–
Gendel	1974	51	–	–	< 1	–
		89[10]	no increase over controls			
Chlorpromazine						
Cohen et al.	1967a	3	9–30	700	10.6	4.0–17.4
Cohen et al.	1969	6	26–54	533	2.8	1.3–4.0
Nielsen et al.	1969	13[6]	–	794	1.9	–
Jenkins	1970	3[11]	17–28	278	27.7	16.9–35.4
Gilmour et al.	1971	11	–	600	2.0[3]	–
Cohen et al.	1972	10	23–63	–	1.1[8]	1.0–1.2
Perphenazine						
Nielsen et al.	1969	15[12]	–	1,047	3.8	–
Cohen et al.	1972	9	23–63	–	1.3[8]	1.2–1.4
Lithium						
Friedrich and Nielsen	1969	3	45–70	215	5.1	1.6–8.6
Jarvik et al.	1971	16	30–64	1,433	3.3	0–12.0

1 Light users.
2 Heavy users ± LSD.
3 Percent cells with breaks.
4 Light and heavy users.
5 Percent cells with breaks and gaps.
6 48-hour cultures.
7 72-hour cultures.

Table V (continued)

Author	Year	Controls				
		subjects	age range years	cells analyzed	mean % breaks	range
Marijuana						
Dorrance et al.	1970	10	18–44	1,018	0.8	0–2.0
Gilmour et al.	1971	16	–	771	0.5[3]	–
Rubin et al.	1973	30	–	–	2.9[5]	–
Stenchever et al.	1974	20	13–52	2,000	1.2[3]	0–5.0
Opiates						
Gilmour et al.	1971	16	–	771	0.5[3]	
Falek et al.	1972	16	21–40	728	0.1	–
		16	21–40	771	0.4	–
Falek and McFadden	1973	13	21–29	728	3.2[9]	0–8.9
Abrams and Liao	1974	14	–	1,400	1.4	–
Gendel	1974	40	–	–	< 1	–
		48	–	–	–	–
Chlorpromazine						
Cohen et al.	1967a	12	22–59	2,674	3.8	2.0–5.5
Cohen et al.	1969	6	21–61	579	2.9	1.3–4.0
Nielsen et al.	1969	41	–	1,584	0.3	–
Jenkins	1970	4	20–30	308	10.1	8.2–14.1
Gilmour et al.	1971	16	–	771	0.5[3]	–
Cohen et al.	1972	10	23–63	–	1.5[9]	1.5–1.6
		6	–	–	1.3	0.5–2.0
Perphenazine						
Nielsen et al.	1969	41	–	1,584	0.3	–
Cohen et al.	1972	9	23–63	–	1.8[9]	1.5–2.1
		6	–	–	1.3	0.5–2.0
Lithium						
Friedrich and Nielsen	1969	11	67 ± 8.8	554	0.5	–
Jarvik et al.	1971	10[13]	33–73	850	1.5	0–6.0
		4[14]	34–73	320	0.9	0–2.0

8 Average of all postdrug values.
9 Average of washout and baseline values.
10 *In utero* exposure to heroin.
11 Also on stelazine.
12 Also on orphenadrine.
13 Drug-free controls.
14 Patients on placebo.

Table V (continued)

Author	Year	Users				
		subjects	age range years	cells analyzed	mean % breaks	range
Chlordiazepoxide *Cohen et al.*	1969	4	46−57	303	3.0	0−9.1
		6	−	1,720	3.0	1.0−7.0
Diazepam *Cohen et al.*	1969	6	12−24	555	2.9	1.0−5.1
Fluphenazine *Cohen et al.*	1969	3	31−44	296	4.4	3.0−7.0
Thioridazine *Cohen et al.*	1969	3	29−52	297	3.0	1.0−4.1

1 Light users.
2 Heavy users ± LSD.
3 Percent cells with breaks.
4 Light and heavy users.
5 Percent cells with breaks and gaps.
6 48-hour cultures.
7 72-hour cultures.

Marijuana

Human Studies

In vivo. There are four reports on chromosome examinations in marijuana users (table V). *Gilmour et al.* (1971) found a higher frequency of chromosome aberrations in eleven heavy users of marijuana, some of whom had also taken LSD, compared to 16 nonusers. However, no increase was seen in a group of 13 light users. *Stenchever et al.* (1974) confirmed an increase in chromosome breakage in 49 users in comparison to 20 controls. The remaining two studies, one by *Dorrance et al.* (1970) and a preliminary report on a clinical study conducted in Jamaica (*Rubin et al.,* 1973), gave negative results. In the Jamaican study, none of the subjects used any other drug.

On the basis of our own prospective study with chromosome examinations prior to, at weekly intervals during, and at 1 month after controlled marijuana use, we are unable to make a definitive statement concerning the chromosome-damaging potential of marijuana (*Matsuyama et al.,* in preparation). In this study, male subjects smoked marijuana under close supervision while confined to

Table V (continued)

Author	Year	Controls				
		subjects	age range years	cells analyzed	mean % breaks	range
Chlordiazepoxide						
Cohen et al.	1969	4	42–63	302	3.6	1.4–6.0
		6	–	1,798	3.4	0.0–7.0
Diazepam						
Cohen et al.	1969	6	14–19	473	2.5	1.4–4.7
Fluphenazine						
Cohen et al.	1969	6	21–61	579	2.9	1.3–4.0
Thioridazine						
Cohen et al.	1969	6	21–61	579	2.9	1.3–4.0

8 Average of all postdrug values.
9 Average of washout and baseline values.
10 *In utero* exposure to heroin.
11 Also on stelazine.
12 Also on orphenadrine.
13 Drug-free controls.
14 Patients on placebo.

a psychiatric ward for the duration of testing. Recently, *Nahas et al.* (1974) reported that 51 chronic marijuana smokers showed a significantly reduced responsiveness to phytohemagglutinin and leukocytes as compared to 80 'normal' individuals, and concluded that marijuana impairs cell-mediated immune reactions. Further studies with matched controls are required to confirm this finding. The relevance of immune changes to cytogenetic analysis rests in the fact that the cells showing reduced responsiveness in the above experiments are also the cells analyzed in the usual chromosome studies.

In vitro. Tetrahydrocannabinol, presumably the most relevant component of marijuana, has been studied *in vitro* (table VI). *Neu et al.* (1970) reported that Δ^8-THC, added to leukocyte cultures during the final 24 h of culture decreased the mitotic index with increasing concentrations but did not increase the number of breaks above that found in control cultures. No structural rearrangements were seen. Preliminary studies with Δ^9-THC yielded similar results. *Stenchever and Allen* (1972) also reported negative results with Δ^9-THC. By contrast, *Leuchtenberger et al.* (1973) reported that human lung explants ex-

Table VI. Reports of chromosome analyses on *in vitro* addition of drugs

Author	Year	No drug added			Drug added			dosage	duration, h
		cells analyzed	mean % breaks	range	cells analyzed	mean % breaks	range		
Marijuana									
Neu et al.[1]	1970	–	<5		–	<5	–	30, 35, 40, 45 µg/ml	24
Stenchever and Allen	1972	903	2.7	1.5–5.5	2,738	1.7	0–3.9	100, 10, 1, 0.1 µg/ml	72
Methadone									
Falek et al.	1972	no significant difference from treated values			450[2]	1.8	1.3–2.7	3 ×, 1 ×, 1/3 ×, 1/6 ×, 1/12 × 0.013 µg/ml	4, 24, 48
Morphine									
Falek et al.	1972	no breaks at all concentrations at all time intervals						3 ×, 1 ×, 1/3 ×, 1/6 ×, 1/12 × 0.002 µg/ml	4, 24, 48
Chlorpromazine									
Abdullah and Miller	1968	100	0	–	100	8.0	–	$8 \times 10^{-6} M$	48
Cohen et al.	1969	–	0.8	–	–	0–2.5	–	100, 10, 1 µg/ml[3]	6, 24, 48
Kamada et al.	1971	500	0.8[4]	–	1,436	1.1[4]	0.7–1.4	$5 \times 10^{-5}, 2 \times 10^{-5}, 10^{-5}, 2 \times 10^{-6} M$	72
					2,500	1.0[4]	0.6–1.2	$2 \times 10^{-5} M$	24, 42, 54, 68, 72
Lithium									
Friedrich and Nielsen	1969	473	–	–	477	no significant increase over controls		1.2, 1.8, 2.4 mEq/l	48

	Year								
Meprobamate									
Kamada et al.	1971	500	0.6[4]	—	1,500	0.8[4]	0.6–1.0	$10^{-4}, 5 \times 10^{-4},$ $10^{-5} M$	72
					1,500	1.0[4]	1.0	$10^{-3} M$	24, 54, 72
Chlordiazepoxide									
Staiger	1969	602[5]	6.6	4.0–10.0	901[5]	7.3	1.0–17.0	50–200 μg/ml	8–72
Diazepam									
Staiger	1969	500[5]	9.2	6.0–14.0	800[5]	6.8	4.0–13.0	12.5–50 μg/ml	8–96
Stenchever and Frankel	1969	700	3.9	1.5–4.8	1,400	15.3[4]	3.0–22.2	20, 10, 1.0, 0. μg/ml	72
Staiger	1970	600[6]	4.0	1.0–10.0	793[6]	4.2	0–11.0	12.5–50 μg/ml	8–96
		800[7]	9.1	5.0–21.0	800[7]	7.1	4.0–12.0	10–40 μg/ml	72

1 Δ^{8}-THC added.
2 Cord blood used.
3 10 and 1 mg cytotoxic.
4 Percent abnormal cells.
5 Human diploid fibroblast cell lines.
6 Whole blood.
7 Separated leukocytes.

posed to marijuana smoke showed variability in DNA content (measured by Feulgen microfluorometry) and chromosome numbers greater than those seen in controls, suggesting an alteration of chromosomal complements.

Animal Studies

Martin (1969) reported on the effects of cannabis resin on chromosomes from cultured rat leukocytes, rat embryonic cells in tissue culture, and cells cultured from rat embryos of mothers treated with a teratogenic dose. She found no increase in breaks when compared to controls, but did find a decrease in mitotic activity with increasing concentrations.

Opiates

Human Studies

In vivo. Heroin and methadone have been studied *in vivo* (table V). *Gilmour et al.* (1971) showed an increase in the percent of cells with one or more aberrations in heroin users as compared to controls. In a study of 16 opiate addicts on methadone maintenance, *Falek et al.* (1972) found a significant increase in chromosome aberrations after 72 h of culture, but not after 48 h of culture. In a follow-up study (*Falek and McFadden,* 1973), serial determinations were carried out on 13 subjects on methadone. The frequency of breaks in predrug leukocyte cultures was 3.2 % compared to 5.0 % at 24 h postdrug (ten subjects). At 8, 20, and 30 weeks of maintenance, the values were 3.9, 4.8, and 4.2 %, respectively, and the mean percent breaks for all postdrug cultures was 4.5 %, a small but statistically significant increase over controls. However, *Gendel* (1974) found less than 1 % breaks in both 40 control mothers and 51 mothers addicted to heroin or methadone.

In utero. Abrams and Liao (1974) studied 16 newborn infants of mothers who used heroin during pregnancy and 14 newborn infants of non-drug-using mothers. They reported a 1.4 % frequency of chromosome breaks in controls, and a significantly elevated frequency of 11.4 % for heroin-exposed infants including a large number of structural abnormalities in contrast to controls where none was seen. *Gendel* (1974) again failed to find an increased frequency of breaks (89 newborn infants of addicted mothers in comparison to the 48 newborn controls). *Zelson et al.* (1971) reported that 4 of 384 infants born to heroin-addicted mothers were born with congenital anomalies, an incidence similar to that found in the general newborn population.

In vitro. In an attempt to determine if methadone was responsible for the elevated rate of breaks seen in their *in vivo* study, *Falek et al.* (1972) tested methadone, morphine, and quinine *in vitro* (table VI). At different concentrations (based on established therapeutic doses) and various durations of exposure, none of these agents showed an increase in breaks.

Chlorpromazine (Thorazine)

Human Studies

In vivo. There are six reports in the literature on the effects of therapeutically administered chlorpromazine, three of which originated from the laboratory of Dr. *M. Cohen* (table V). In the first report (*Cohen et al.,* 1967a) an increased frequency of breaks was found when compared to controls. However, in a subsequent investigation of an additional six subjects, no increase was seen (*Cohen et al.,* 1969). *Nielsen et al.* (1969) and *Gilmour et al.* (1971) did find an increase in the frequency of breaks in patients treated with chlorpromazine when compared to control subjects as did *Jenkins* (1970) despite an unusually high control value (10.1 %). All of the subjects in *Jenkins'* study were also on stelazine. In a well-designed prospective study by *Cohen et al.* (1972) with chromosome examinations prior to, during, and following chlorpromazine treatment of ten patients, no increase in breaks was found. Values after 3 and 6 weeks of treatment, and at a 1-month follow-up were compared to baseline values. Six control subjects were also studied in parallel and no differences were found.

In vitro. In addition to the above *in vivo* studies, there are three studies of *in vitro* effects (table VI). *Abdullah and Miller* (1968) found an increased frequency of breaks when chlorpromazine was added to fibroblast cultures at a concentration of $8 \times 10^{-6}M$ (8 vs. 0 %). At a higher concentration of $8 \times 10^{-5}M$, no mitoses were seen. In a second experiment, fibroblast cultures from another individual were utilized, and again an increase was found (5 vs. 1 %). *Cohen et al.* (1969) added chlorpromazine (10 and 1 mg/ml, 100, 10 and 1 μg/ml) at 48, 24, and 6 h prior to harvest, and found that at concentrations of 1 and 10 mg/ml no metaphases were seen. For 1, 10, and 100 μg/ml, there was significant mitotic inhibition, and this effect was related to duration of exposure. However, at concentrations where cells for chromosome analyses were available, no increased damage was observed. *Kamada et al.* (1971) were also unable to demonstrate any chromosome-damaging effect following *in vitro* addition of chlorpromazine to lymphocyte cultures.

Animal Studies

Siva Sankar and Geisler (1971) administered chlorpromazine intravenously to mice, and blood for analysis was drawn 1 and 24 h later. At 1 h, a cytotoxic effect was seen with very few metaphases available for examination. At 24 h there was no effect on growth, but a significant increase in total breaks was found. *Kelly-Garvert and Legator* (1973) designed an *in vitro* experiment on a Chinese hamster cell line based on the report that chlorpromazine forms stable ions when photoactivated with UV light. It is postulated that these radicals in turn intercalate into DNA, causing damage. Chlorpromazine, to give a final concentration of 3.5 mg/ml, was added to cultures and exposed to dark light for 0–10 min. They found an increasing frequency of cells with rearrangements with increasing duration of exposure to light.

Perphenazine (Trilafon)

Human Studies
In vivo. There are two reports on the cytogenetic effects of perphenazine (table V). In the first report, *Nielsen et al.* (1969) found a significantly higher frequency of breaks in those individuals taking perphenazine as compared to age-matched controls. However, these patients were also given orphenadrine (Disipal), and there is the possibility that this increase may be due to the synergistic effects of orphenadrine and perphenazine. Two additional cases with chromosome analyses prior to, and twice during treatment, also showed an increase in breaks. However, in a recent prospective study (*Cohen et al.,* 1972) where individuals served as their own control with two chromosome examinations prior to drug administration, one at 3- and one at 6-week intervals during treatment, and one at a 1-month follow-up, no increase in the frequency of breaks could be demonstrated.

Lithium

Human Studies
In vivo. There are two cytogenetic studies on lithium (table V). *Friedrich and Nielsen* (1969) found a significantly higher frequency of breaks and hypo-diploid cells in three psychiatric patients on lithium therapy than in age-matched controls. In the study by *Jarvik et al.* (1971) the 16 patients on lithium also showed a higher frequency of breaks but the difference was not statistically significant when compared with drug-free controls. However, the placebo group had significantly fewer breaks than the lithium-treated patients. These findings must be interpreted with caution since five of the lithium patients were also receiving other drugs and their mean break frequency was 4.5 % compared to only 2.7 % for the remaining eleven patients on lithium alone.

In utero. While no chromosome data are available on infants exposed *in utero, Schou and Amdisen* (1970) reported that of 40 mothers on lithium therapy during pregnancy, two gave birth to children with malformations. Unfortunately, there are no comparative malformation rates for the offspring of psychiatric patients not on lithium.

In vitro. Friedrich and Nielsen (1969) carried out *in vitro* studies on leukocyte cultures (table VI). Lithium at doses approximating serum concentrations added for the duration of culture (48 h) did not increase the frequency of breaks when compared to control cultures.

Animal Studies
Szabo (1970) reported palatal defects and increased fetal resorption in mice following oral administration of lithium, and believes lithium to be selective for palatal development since ear and eye defects were not seen. Two studies on rats (*Trautner et al.*, 1958; *Johansen and Ulrich*, 1969) failed to demonstrate a teratogenic effect following oral administration. In contrast, *Wright et al.* (1971) observed increased resorption rates and cranial malformations in the fetuses of rats given lithium intraperitoneally during pregnancy, and postulates that the route of administration may be responsible for the differing results.

Chlordiazepoxide (Librium)

Human Studies
In vivo. Cohen et al. (1969) studied four subjects on chlordiazepoxide and four controls, and found no increase in breaks (table V). In addition, serial determinations were done on six subjects given the drug and six controls at 2-week intervals during an 8-week period, and no increase in breaks or structural abnormalities was observed.

In vitro. An *in vitro* study by *Staiger* (1969) on human fibroblasts gave negative results (table VI). Concentrations used were 25–100 times higher than the blood level of 2 μg/ml obtained 2–4 h following a single oral dose of 30 mg.

Animal Studies
Schmid and Staiger (1969) studied the *in vivo* effect on Chinese hamsters following oral administration. Again the results were negative.

Diazepam (Valium)

Human Studies
In vivo. Cohen et al. (1969) studied six patients who had been on diazepam for 3–6 years and did not find an increased incidence of chromosome damage in comparison to controls (table V).

In utero. There are two case reports of congenital abnormalities in infants born to mothers who had received diazepam during their pregnancies (*Istvan,* 1970; *Ringrose,* 1972). Although the duration is not stated, it is known that in both cases diazepam was taken at least during the first trimester. However, other drugs were also taken during this period, in one case propoxyphene HCl (Darvon 65) as necessary for headaches, and in the other hydroxyprogesterone (Delalutin) over a prolonged period of time. The significance, if any, of isolated case reports must be carefully weighed due to the reporting bias.

In vitro. There are three reports on the *in vitro* effects of diazepam (table VI). For purposes of comparison with *in vivo* blood levels, it should be noted that a blood level of 1 μg/ml of diazepam is obtained following repeated daily doses of 30 mg (*de Silva et al.,* 1966). At concentrations 12–50 times higher than blood levels, *Staiger* (1969) found no increase in breaks or structural abnormalities in three different human diploid fibroblast cell lines. In 1970, *Staiger* investigated the effects on human lymphocytes, utilizing similar concentrations and two different culture techniques, but could not demonstrate any effect. In contrast to the above, using a wide range of concentrations including those reported to be within the therapeutic range, *Stenchever and Frankel* (1969) did show a dose-dependent increase in the number of cells with breaks. No structural abnormalities were seen; the increase was accounted for by chromatid and chromosome breaks exclusively.

Animal Studies

Schmid and Staiger (1969) examined bone marrow chromosomes of Chinese hamsters following oral administration (19 doses of 300 and 900 mg/kg), and found no increase in breaks or structural abnormalities. *Beall* (1972) tested the teratogenic potential of diazepam on rats. No effect on the number of pregnant rats, number of resorptions, and average litter size was seen; nor was the drug found to be teratogenic.

Other Psychotherapeutic Agents

Cohen et al. (1969) reported negative results for fluphenazine (Prolixin, Permitil) and thioridazine (Mellaril) (table V). However, these findings are based on a limited number of subjects (three in each group).

In vitro addition of various concentrations of meprobamate (Miltown) to leukocyte cultures and for different durations of exposure also gave negative results (*Kamada et al.,* 1971) (table VI). *Jagiello et al.* (1973) conducted *in vivo* and *in vitro* meiotic cytogenetic studies with meprobamate in mice. *In vitro* concentrations tested on mouse ova ranged from 1 to 10,000 μg/ml. At

750 µg/ml, meiotic processes were halted while at 500 µg/ml an increase in abnormal second metaphase figures was seen. However, acute or chronic *in vivo* treatment of mice had no effect on meiosis.

Bone marrow examinations of Chinese hamsters following oral administration of medazepam (Nobrium, ten doses of 450 mg/kg) showed no increase in breaks (*Schmid and Staiger, 1969*).

Imipramine (Tofranil) is considered teratogenic in man (*McBride, 1972*), yet *Levy* (1972) states that he has successfully treated 'hundreds of patients, many of whom were pregnant' without side effects. *Gilani* (1974) injected chick eggs with imipramine and found extensive toxic effects on developing chick embryos. *In vitro* addition of imipramine at different concentrations and for different durations decreased the number of mitoses, an index of cell division (*Fu et al.,* 1973). This effect was time and dose dependent.

Recently, cytogenetic and teratogenic effects of anticonvulsants have been studied. *Zellweger* (1974), in reviewing the literature, found a high incidence of tetraploid cells in four of six children exposed *in utero.* The significance of this finding, however, is unclear. Mention is also made of five additional children exposed *in utero,* and their mothers, all of whom manifested structural abnormalities (including chromosome breaks, triradial and quadriradial rearrangements). With regard to teratogenesis, *South* (1972), in a review of the literature, found a high incidence of congenital abnormalities in the offspring of 677 epileptic women on drugs during pregnancy as compared to no abnormalities in 201 epileptic women not on drugs.

Discussion and Conclusion

In recent years, there has been a tremendous upsurge of interest in the harmful effects of drugs on chromosomes. The research has elicited contradictory information which only adds to the seriousness of the situation, especially since greater numbers of people are continually becoming exposed to drugs.

In areas of medicine where drugs are life preserving, possible deleterious side effects, including genetic damage, are a necessary evil. In the treatment of mental disorders, however, the same risks need not be taken. Numerous psychoactive agents as well as alternate forms of therapy are available. Moreover, the accesibility of drugs to seemingly healthy people who use them for relatively minor complaints, further increases the number of persons exposed to possible genetic damage from psychoactive agents. It is of particular importance, therefore, that we have knowledge of the risk of genetic damage accompanying the use of psychoactive agents whether used therapeutically or abused.

Aside from the direct risk of genetic damage another far reaching consequence of modern pharmacotherapy is to reduce the length of hospitalization of individuals undergoing treatment. In schizophrenia, for example, the result is an increased opportunity to procreate, leading to an increased reproductive rate in these patients (*Erlenmeyer-Kimling et al.,* 1969). This, in turn, causes a re-structuring of the gene pool with the potential not only of increasing the number of individuals predisposed to schizophrenia but conceivably, as a result of pharmacotherapy, also those predisposed to malignant neoplasia and congenital anomalies.

In addition to the foregoing considerations there is, of course, the major problem presented by the increasing numbers of drug abusers in our present society who consist primarily of young persons still in their childbearing years.

Unfortunately, we lack precise information regarding the significance of chromosome breaks. If knowledge is lacking on the mutagenic and carcinogenic potential of these drugs, even less is known about their teratogenic potential. This survey has not attempted to include a thorough review of the latter, although an attempt has been made to include all available information on the former.

Cytogenetic studies have been carried out *in vivo* and *in vitro* on humans and animals. Human and animal studies have also been done *in utero,* but frequently two critical factors, the time and route of administration of the drugs, have not been mentioned, presenting difficulty in accurately evaluating the results.

There are numerous problems inherent in cytogenetic assessment of drug effects. Leukocyte cells from blood samples have been used almost exclusively because they are readily obtained, but these are not gonadal cells and inferences have to be made that changes in one cellular system reflect those in another when extrapolating from peripheral leukocytes to congenital malformations. In addition there is the problem that *in vivo* and *in vitro* findings do not always correspond.

Cytogenetic results may be influenced by a number of factors. Deficiencies in culture media (*Sparkes et al.,* 1968; *Freed and Schatz,* 1969), the source of leukocytes (whether cord, venous, or capillary blood), individual differences, and seasonal variation, have been proposed as explanations for the discrepant findings from study to study. Recent viral infections and radiation exposures of individuals whose cells are cultured represent another uncontrolled source of variability. Indeed, because of high aberration frequencies, some investigators have eliminated from their control groups individuals with a history of either of the latter. Observer scoring of aberrations may be yet another factor, particularly in light of the relative consistency with which positive and negative results emanate from the same laboratories. Finally, the tediousness of cytogenetic analysis allows for only a small number of individuals to be examined. All of the above interfere with gaining a clear picture of chromosome damage ascribable to any one drug.

A few investigators reporting negative results have been critical of the unusually elevated frequency of chromosome aberrations in control groups of positive studies. However, even in normal populations, there have been wide variations in the frequency with which aberrations have been reported, although basically the same techniques have been utilized in all laboratories. *Bloom and Tjio* (1964) reported no breaks in 20 subjects, while *Schmickel* (1967) found a frequency of 0.7 % in eleven subjects. In two large studies, *Court Brown et al.* (1966) and *Sandberg et al.* (1967) reported mean break frequencies of 0.4 and 1.7 %, respectively.

In contrast to the above studies, *Lubs and Samuelson* (1967) analyzed ten subjects and found a mean break frequency of 7.4 %. *Littlefield and Goh* (1973) reported their findings on serial determinations conducted on 31 subjects, ten men and 21 women. A total of 29,709 metaphases from 305 cultures were analyzed with a frequency of 7.1 %. Women showed considerably more variability from culture to culture and a higher frequency than men (7.6 and 6.4 %, respectively). For both men and women, a significantly increased overall frequency of breaks was found during the late spring and early summer months, as contrasted to other times of the year. The report of seasonal variation needs further investigation. For example, if drug users are more susceptible to viral infections, then studies conducted during a flu epidemic may show a significant increase in breaks unrelated to the drug under study. Despite such marked discrepancies, *Jarvik and Yen* (1974) reported that chromosome examinations done 2 years apart on seven individuals yielded nearly identical mean break frequencies (although there was considerable individual variability).

One new approach to the study of drug effects concentrates on cellular proliferation in response to mitogens (agents stimulating cell division). Response is measured by comparing the level of incorporation of DNA-specific radioactive thymidine into cells prior to, and following, acute administration of the drug in question, or by comparing responses of chronic drug users to responses of matched controls. However, it must be pointed out that there is no perfect correlation between response to mitogens and chromosome damage. Some drugs may have no effect on cell proliferation but are capable of producing extensive chromosome damage while other drugs may reduce cell proliferation without producing an increased frequency of chromosome damage (marijuana, according to *Neu et al.*, 1970; imipramine, according to *Fu et al.*, 1973; and chlorpromazine, according to *Cohen et al.*, 1969). Therefore, although the procedure returns a quick dividend, it does not appear to be sufficient to exonerate any drug from having potentially deleterious effects.

Certain limitations were generally encountered in attempting to evaluate the findings in the literature. They included lack of proper controls, inadequate sample sizes (some reports are based on one or two individuals), unknown composition of 'street' drugs (see section on LSD for example), scarcity of information on health care and socioeconomic status of the subjects, insufficient data on exogenous agents (i.e. exposure to other drugs including caffeine, chemicals, radiation, and viral infections, all of which are known to be mutagenic agents), paucity of chromosome analyses before, during, and after administration of drugs, and lack of follow-up studies. Many, if not all of these, may contribute to the increased frequency of chromosome damage reported for drug 'users'. On the other hand, it is conceivable that these limitations may have prevented the surfacing of even more incriminating data.

The possibility of individual differences in susceptibility to chromosome damage must also be considered. Although the basic components of DNA are identical in all individuals, heterozygosity prevails and may characterize as much as 20 % of genetic loci in man (*Harris and Hopkinson*, 1972). Hence, the well-known existence of interindividual variability at the biochemical level. Even if pathways of drug metabolism are similar, the rates of metabolism may differ markedly, and equivalent dosages may not necessarily mean equal serum levels. Genetic factors have been shown to play prominent roles in determining serum concentrations for nortryptiline (*Alexanderson et al.*, 1969) and alcohol (*Vesell et al.*, 1971). (For a more thorough discussion, see *Propping and Kopun*, 1973.) Thus, interindividual differences may operate at several levels to produce differences in susceptibility to chromosome damage. Nonetheless, most of the publications have ignored such differences.

In the light of the above, it is not surprising that the literature reviewed yielded few clear-cut conclusions. These may be summarized as follows:

LSD. In vitro addition of LSD to leukocyte cultures produces an increase in chromosome damage which is *not* dose dependent. *In vivo* studies of LSD users, persons given LSD under medical supervision, and infants exposed *in utero,* have been contradictory, some reporting increased damage, others not. No relationship has been found between dosage and/or duration of exposure and frequency of chromosome aberrations. In some studies, those individuals having used LSD the longest were among those showing the lowest frequency of breaks. The majority of the studies have been retrospective. The few well-controlled prospective studies with chromosome analyses prior to, during, and after drug administration failed to detect a significant effect of LSD on chromosomes.

Marijuana. Reports are contradictory, except that 'users' of 'street' drugs usually show increased frequency of breaks.

Other drugs. Data are insufficient for any summary statement at this time. There is further need for cytogenetic analyses to test the potentially harmful effects of drugs on the genetic material of man. Such studies should be carefully designed and include samples of adequate size with chromosome examinations prior to, during, and at intervals following treatment. However, the requirement for highly skilled individuals to conduct the chromosome examinations, and the time-consuming nature of this type of study are distinct disadvantages of the method. It is hoped that these disadvantages will be overcome once computer-aided analysis has been developed into a routine procedure.

In the meantime, however, the data are such as to preclude complacency until more definitive information is acquired.

References

Aase, J.M.; Laestadius, N., and Smith, D.W.: Children of mothers who took LSD in pregnancy. Lancet *ii:* 100–101 (1970).

Abbo, G.; Norris, A., and Zellweger, H.: Lysergic acid diethylamide (LSD-25) and chromosome breaks. Humangenetik *6:* 253–258 (1968).

Abdullah, S. and Miller, O.J.: Effect of drugs on nucleic acid synthesis and cell division *in vitro.* Dis. nerv. Syst. *29:* 829–833 (1968).

Abrams, C.A.L. and Liao, P.Y.: A look at heroin's cytotoxic potential. Lab. Mgmt *12:* 10–12 (1974).

Alexanderson, B.; Price Evans, D.A., and Sjöqvist, F.: Steady-state plasma levels of nortriptyline in twins. Influence of genetic factors and drug therapy. Brit. med. J. *iv:* 764–768 (1969).

Anonymous: Hallucinogen and teratogen? Lancet *ii:* 504–505 (1967).

Assemany, S.R.; Neu, R.L., and Gardner, L.I.: Deformities in a child whose mother took LSD. Lancet *i:* 1290 (1970).

Beall, J.R.: Study of the teratogenic potential of diazepam and SCH 12041. Canad. med. Ass. J. *106:* 1061 (1972).

Bender, L. and Siva Sankar, D.V.: Chromosome damage not found in leukocytes of children treated with LSD-25. Science *159:* 749 (1968).

Bick, Y.A.E.: Comparison of the effects of LSD, heliotrine and X-irradiation on chromosome breakage, and the effects of LSD on the rate of cell division. Nature, Lond. *226:* 1165–1167 (1970).

Bloom, A.D. and Tjio, J.H.: In vivo effect of diagnostic X-irradiation on human chromosomes. New Engl. J. Med. *270:* 1341–1344 (1964).

Browning, L.S.: Lysergic acid diethylamide. Mutagenic effects in *Drosophila.* Science *161:* 1022–1023 (1968).

Carakushansky, G.; Neu, R.L., and Gardner, L.I.: Lysergide and cannabis as possible teratogens in man. Lancet *ii:* 150–151 (1969).

Cohen, M.M.; Hirschhorn, K., and Frosch, W.A.: In vivo and in vitro chromosomal damage induced by LSD-25. New Engl. J. Med. *277:* 1043–1049 (1967a).

Cohen, M.M.; Hirschhorn, K., and Frosch, W.A.: Cytogenetic effects of tranquilizing drugs in vivo and in vitro. J. amer. med. Ass. *207:* 2425–2426 (1969).

Cohen, M.M.; Hirschhorn, K.; Verbo, S.; Frosch, W.A., and Groeschel, M.M.: The effect of LSD-25 on the chromosomes of children exposed in utero. Pediatrics *2:* 486–492 (1968).

Cohen, M.M.; Leiber, E., and Schwartz, H.N.: In vivo cytogenetic effects of perphenazine and chlorpromazine. A negative study. Brit. med. J. *iii:* 21–23 (1972).

Cohen, M.M.; Marinello, M.J., and Back, N.: Chromosomal damage in human leukocytes induced by lysergic acid diethylamide. Science *155:* 1417–1419 (1967b).

Cohen, M.M. and Mukherjee, A.B.: Meiotic chromosome damage induced by LSD-25. Nature, Lond. *219:* 1072–1074 (1968).

Corey, M.J.; Andrews, J.C.; McLeod, M.J.; MacLean, J.R., and Wilby, W.E.: Chromosome studies on patients *(in vivo)* and cells *(in vitro)* treated with lysergic acid diethylamide. New Engl. J. Med. *282:* 939–943 (1970).

Court Brown, W.M.; Buckton, K.E.; Jacobs, P.A.; Tough, M.; Kuenssberg, E.V., and Knox, J.D.E.: Chromosome studies on adults. Eugenics Laboratory Memoirs No. 42 (Cambridge University Press, London 1966).

Dishotsky, N.I.; Loughman, W.D.; Mogar, R.E., and Lipscomb, W.R.: LSD and genetic damage. Science *172:* 431–440 (1971).

Dorrance, D.; Janiger, O., and Teplitz, R.L.: In vivo effects of illicit hallucinogens on human lymphocyte chromosomes. J. amer. med. Ass. *212:* 1488–1491 (1970).

Dumars, K.W.: Parental drug usage. Effect upon chromosomes of progeny. Pediatrics *47:* 1037–1041 (1971).

Egozcue, J. and Irwin, S.: Effect of LSD-25 on mitotic and meiotic chromosomes of mice and monkey. Humangenetik *8:* 86–93 (1969).

Egozcue, J.; Irwin, S., and Maruffo, C.A.: Chromosomal damage in LSD users. J. amer. med. Ass. *204:* 122–126 (1968).

Eller, J.L. and Morton, J.M.: Bizarre deformities in offspring of users of lysergic acid diethylamide. New Engl. J. Med. *283:* 395–397 (1970).

Emerit, I.; Roux, C., and Feingold, J.: LSD. No chromosomal breakage in mother and embryos during rat pregnancy. Teratology *6:* 71–74 (1972).

Erlenmeyer-Kimling, L.; Nicol, S.; Rainer, J.D., and Deming, W.E.: Changes in fertility rates of schizophrenic patients in New York state. Amer. J. Psychiat. *125:* 88–99 (1969).

Falek, A.; Jordan, R.B.; King, B.J.; Arnold, P.J., and Skelton, W.D.: Human chromosomes and opiates. Arch. gen. Psychiat. *27:* 511–515 (1972).

Falek, A. and McFadden, I.J.: Cytogenetic follow-up of patients in a methadone maintenance program – a pilot study. Proc. 5th Nat. Conf. on Methadone Treatment, Washington 1973, pp. 695–705.

Fernandez, J.; Browne, I.W.; Cullen, J.; Brennan, T.; Matheu, H.; Fischer, I.; Masterson, J., and Law, E.: LSD ... an *in vivo* retrospective chromosome study. Ann. hum. Genet. *37:* 81–91 (1973).

Fischer, P.; Golob, E.; Kunze-Muehl, E., and Muellner, T.: Chromosome aberrations in persons with thorium dioxide burdens; in *Evans, Court Brown and McLean* Human radiation cytogenetics, pp. 194–202 (1967).

Freed, J.J. and Schatz, S.A.: Chromosome aberrations in cultured cells deprived of single essential amino acids. Exp. Cell Res. *55:* 393–409 (1969).

Friedrich, U. and Nielsen, J.: Lithium and chromosome abnormalities. Lancet *ii:* 435–436 (1969).

Fu, T.K.; Yen, F.S.; Jarvik, L.F.; Malitz, S., and Glassman, A.: Imipramine and human chromosomes. Genetics *74:* 586 (1973).

Gelhrter, T.D.: Lysergic acid diethylamide (LSD) and exstrophy of the bladder. J. Pediat. *77:* 1065–1066 (1970).

Gendel, E.: Cytotoxic potential of opiates. Lab. Mgmt *12:* 8 (1974).

Genest, P.: Etude cytogénétique des hallucinogènes. Essai préliminaire de la lysergamide (LSD-25) sur la culture des leucocytes humains. Laval méd. *40:* 56–58 (1969).

German, J.: Bloom's syndrome. I. Genetical and clinical observations in the first twenty-seven patients. Amer. J. hum. Genet. *21:* 196–227 (1969).

Gilani, S.H.: Imipramine and congenital abnormalities. Path. Microbiol. *40:* 37–42 (1974).

Gilmour, D.G.; Bloom, A.D.; Lele, K.P.; Robbins, E.S., and Maximillian, C.: Chromosomal aberrations in users of psychoactive drugs. Arch. gen. Psychiat. *24:* 268–272 (1971).

Goetz, P.; Sram, R.J., and Zudova, A.: Effect of LSD on meiotic chromosomes of rat males. Mamm. Chrom. Newsl. *13:* 114–117 (1972).

Grace, D.; Carlson, E.A., and Goodman, P.: Drosophila melanogaster treated with LSD. Absence of mutations and chromosome breakage. Science *161:* 694–696 (1968).

Grouchy, J. de: Chromosomes in neoplastic tissues; in *Crow and Neel* Proc. 3rd Int. Congr. Human Genetics, pp. 137–149 (John Hopkins Press, Baltimore 1967).

Harris, H. and Hopkinson, D.A.: Average heterozygosity per locus in man: an estimate based on the incidence of enzyme polymorphisms. Ann. hum. Genet. *36:* 9–20 (1972).

Hecht, F.; Beals, R.K.; Lees, M.H.; Jolly, H., and Roberts, P.: Lysergic acid diethylamide and cannabis as possible teratogens in man. Lancet *ii:* 1087 (1968).

Hirschhorn, K. and Bloch-Shtacher, N.: Transformation of genetically abnormal cells; in Genetic concepts and neoplasia, pp. 191–202 (Williams & Wilkins, Baltimore 1970).

Hsu, L.Y.; Strauss, L., and Hirschhorn, K.: Chromosome abnormality in offspring of LSD user. J. amer. med. Ass. *211:* 987–990 (1970).

Hulten, M.; Lindsten, J.; Lidberg, L., and Ekelund, H.: Studies on mitotic and meiotic chromosomes in subjects exposed to LSD. Ann. Génét. *11:* 201–210 (1968).

Hungerford, D.A.; Taylor, K.M.; Shagass, C.; LaBadie, G.U.; Balaban, G.B., and Paton, G.R.: Cytogenetic effects of LSD-25 therapy in man. J. amer. med. Ass. *206:* 2287–2291 (1968).

Idanpaan-Heikkila, J.E. and Schoolar, J.C.: LSD. Autoradiographic study on the placental tranfer and tissue distribution in mice. Science *164:* 1295–1297 (1969).

Irwin, S. and Egozcue, J.: Chromosomal abnormalities in leukocytes from LSD-25 users. Science *157:* 313–314 (1967).

Istvan, J.: Drug associated congenital abnormalities? Canad. med. Ass. J. *103:* 1394 (1970).

Jacobsen, C.B. and Berlin, C.M.: Possible reproductive detriment in LSD users. J. amer. med. Ass. *222:* 1367–1373 (1972).

Jagiello, G.; Ducayen, M.B., and Lin, J.S.: A meiotic cytogenetic study in mice of a commonly used tranquilizer reported to concentrate in mammalian follicular fluid. Teratology 7: 17–22 (1973).

Jagiello, G. and Polani, P.E.: Mouse germ cells and LSD-25. Cytogenetics *8:* 136–147 (1969).

Jarvik, L.F.; Bishun, N.P.; Bleiweiss, H.; Kato, T., and Moralishvili, E.: Chromosome examinations in patients on lithium carbonate. Arch. gen. Psychiat. *24:* 166–168 (1971).

Jarvik, L.F.; Jaffe, J.; Yen, F.Y.; Kato, T.; Dahlberg, C.C.; Moralishvili, E., and Fleiss, J.L.: Chromosome examinations after medically administered lysergic acid diethylamide and dextroamphetamine. Dis. nerv. Syst. *35:* 399–407 (1974).

Jarvik, L.F.; Kato, T.; Saunders, B., and Moralishvili, E.: LSD and human chromosomes; in *Efron* Psychopharmacology. United States Public Health Service Publication, No. 1836 pp. 1247–1252 (1968).

Jarvik, L.F. and Yen, F.S.: Survival of octogenarians. Six years after initial chromosome examination. 4th Ann. Mtg. Behavior Genetics, Minneapolis 1974.

Jenkins, E.C.: Phenothiazines and chromosome damage. Cytologia *35:* 552–560 (1970).

Johansen, K.T. and Ulrich, K.: Preliminary studies of the possible teratogenic effect of lithium. Acta psychiat. scand., Suppl. 207, pp. 91–95 (1969).

Judd, L.L.; Brandkamp, W.W., and McGlothlin, W.H.: Comparison of the chromosomal patterns obtained from groups of continued users, former users and non-users of LSD-25. Amer. J. Psychiat. *126:* 626–635 (1969).

Kamada, N.; Brecher, G., and Tjio, J.H.: In vitro effects of chlorpromazine and meprobamate on blast transformation and chromosomes. Proc. Soc. exp. Biol. Med. *136:* 210–214 (1971).

Kato, T. and Jarvik, L.F.: LSD-25 and genetic damage. Dis. nerv. Syst. *30:* 42–46 (1969).

Kato, T.; Jarvik, L.F.; Roizin, L., and Moralishvili, E.: Chromosome studies in pregnant Rhesus macaque given LSD-25. Dis. nerv. Syst. *31:* 245–250 (1970).

Kelly-Garvert, F. and Legator, M.S.: Photoactivation of chlorpromazine. Cytogenetic and mutagenic effects. Mutation Res. *21:* 101–105 (1973).

Knudson, A.G.; Strong, L.C., and Anderson, D.E.: Heredity and cancer in man. Progr. med. Genet. *1:* 113–158 (1973).

Krippner, S.: Drug deceptions. Science *168:* 654–655 (1970).

Leuchtenberger, C.; Leuchtenberger, R.; Ritter, U., and Inui, N.: Effects of marijuana and tobacco smoke on DNA and chromosomal complement in human lung explants. Nature, Lond. *242:* 403–404 (1973).

Levy, L.: Imipramine and fetal deformities. Canad. med. Ass. J. *106:* 1057–1058 (1972).

Littlefield, L.G. and Goh, K.O.: Cytogenetic studies in control men and women. I. Variations in aberration frequencies in 29,709 metaphases from 305 cultures obtained over a three-year period. Cytogenet. Cell Genet. *12:* 17–34 (1973).

Loughman, W.D.; Sargent, T.W., and Israelstam, D.M.: Leukocytes of humans exposed to lysergic acid diethylamide: lack of chromosomal damage. Science *158:* 508–510 (1967).

Lubs, H.A. and Samuelson, J.: Chromosome abnormalities in lymphocytes from normal human subjects. Cytogenetics *6:* 402–411 (1967).

Mackenzie, J.B. and Stone, G.E.: Chromosomal abnormalities in human leukocytes exposed to LSD-25 in culture. Mamm. Chrom. Newsl. *9:* 212–216 (1968).

Martin, P.: Cannabis and chromosomes. Lancet *i:* 370 (1969).

McBride, W.G.: The teratogenic effects of imipramine. Teratology *5:* 262 (1972).

McGlothlin, W.H.; Sparkes, R.S., and Arnold, D.O.: Effects of LSD on human pregnancy. J. amer. med. Ass. *212:* 1483–1487 (1970).

Miller, O.J.; Miller, D.A., and Warburton, D.: Application of new staining techniques to the study of human chromosomes. Progr. med. Genet. *9:* 1–48 (1973).

Miller, R.W.: Neoplasia and Down's syndrome. Ann. N.Y. Acad. Sci. *171:* 637–644 (1970).

Moorhead, P.S.; Jarvik, L.F., and Cohen, M.M.: Cytogenetic methods for mutagenicity testing; in *Epstein* Drugs of abuse: their genetic and other chronic nonpsychiatric hazards, pp. 140–170 (MIT Press, Cambridge 1971).

Moorhead, P.S.; Nowell, P.C.; Mellman, W.J.; Battips, D.M., and Hungerford, D.A.: Chromosome preparations of leukocytes cultured from human peripheral blood. Exp. Cell Res. *20:* 613–616 (1960).

Nahas, G.G.; Suciu-Foca, N.; Armand, J.P., and Morishima, A.: Inhibition of cellular mediated immunity in marijuana smokers. Science *183:* 419–420 (1974).

Neu, R.L.; Powers, H.O.; King, S., and Gardner, L.I.: Δ^8- and Δ^9-tetrahydrocannabinol: effects on cultured human leukocytes. J. clin. Pharm. *10:* 228–230 (1970).

Nichols, W.W.: Significance of various type chromosome aberrations for man; in *de Serres and Sheridan* Environmental health perspective experimental issue, No. 6., pp. 179–184 (1973).

Nielsen, J.; Friedrich, U.; Jacobsen, E., and Tsuboi, T.: Lysergide and chromosome abnormalities. Brit. med. J. *ii:* 801–803 (1968).

Nielsen, J.; Friedrich, U., and Tsuboi, T.: Chromosome abnormalities in patients treated with chlorpromazine, perphenazine, and lysergide. Brit. med. J. *iii:* 634–636 (1969).

Propping, P. and Kopun, M.: Pharmacogenetic aspects of psychoactive drugs. Facts and fancy. Humangenetik *20:* 291–320 (1973).

Ringrose, C.A.D.: The hazard of neurotropic drugs in the fertile years. Canad. med. Ass. J. *106:* 1058 (1972).

Rubin, V.; Comitas, L.; Beaubrun, M.H., and Cruickshank, E.K.: No harm found in chronic use of marijuana. Hospital Tribune 7 (35): 1 (1973).

Sandberg, A.A.; Cohen, M.M.; Rimm, A.A., and Levin, M.L.: Aneuploidy and age in a population survey. Amer. J. hum. Genet. *19:* 633–643 (1967).

Sato, H. and Pergament, E.: Is lysergide a teratogen. Lancet *i:* 639–640 (1968).

Sato, H.; Pergament, E., and Nair, V.: LSD in pregnancy. Chromosomal effects. Life Sci. *10:* 773–779 (1971).

Schmickel, R.: Chromosome aberrrations in leukocytes exposed *in vitro* to diagnostic levels of X-rays. Amer. J. hum. Genet. *19:* 1–11 (1967).

Schmid, W. and Staiger, G.R.: Chromosome studies in bone marrow from Chinese hamsters treated with benzodiazepine tranquilizers and cyclophosphamide. Mutation Res. *7:* 99–108 (1969).

Schou, M. and Amdisen, A.: Lithium in pregnancy. Lancet *i:* 1391 (1970).

Silva, J.A.F. de; Koechlin, B.A., and Bader, B.: Blood level distribution patterns of diazepam and its major metabolite in man. J. pharm. Sci. *55:* 692–702 (1966).

Siva Sankar, D.V. and Geisler, A.: Mouse leukocyte chromosome system. Effect of chlorpromazine and aspirin. Res. Commun. chem. Path. Pharmacol. *2:* 477–482 (1971).

Siva Sankar, D.V.; Rozsa, P.W., and Geisler, A.: Chromosome breakage in children treated with LSD-25 and UML-491. Comp. Psychiat. *10:* 406–410 (1969).

Skakkebaek, N.E. and Beatty, R.A.: Studies on meiotic chromosomes and spermatozoan heads in mice treated with LSD. J. Reprod. Fertil. *22:* 141–144 (1970).

Skakkebaek, N.E.; Philip, J., and Rafaelson, O.J.: LSD in mice. Abnormalities in meiotic chromosomes. Science *160:* 1246–1248 (1968).

South, J.: Teratogenic effect of anticonvulsants. Lancet *ii:* 1154 (1972).

Sparkes, R.S.; Melnyk, J., and Bozzeti, L.P.: Chromosomal effect *in vivo* of exposure to lysergic acid diethylamide. Science *160:* 1343–1345 (1968).

Staiger, G.R.: Chlordiazepoxide and diazepam. Absence of effects on the chromosomes of human diploid fibroblast cells. Mutation Res. *7:* 109–115 (1969).

Staiger, G.R.: Studies on the chromosomes of human lymphocytes treated with diazepam *in vitro.* Mutation Res. *10:* 635–644 (1970).

Stenchever, M.A. and Allen, M.: The effect of delta-9-tetrahydrocannabinol on the chromosomes of human lymphocytes *in vitro.* Amer. J. Obstet. Gynec. *114:* 819–821 (1972).

Stenchever, M.A. and Frankel, R.B.: Some effects of diazepam in human cells *in vitro.* Amer. J. Obstet. Gynec. *103:* 836–842 (1969).

Stenchever, M.A. and Jarvis, J.A.: Lysergic acid diethylamide (LSD). Effect on human chromosomes *in vivo.* Amer. J. Obstet. Gynec. *106:* 485–488 (1970).

Stenchever, M.A.; Kunysz, T.J., and Allen, M.A.: Chromosome breakage in users of marijuana. Amer. J. Obstet. Gynec. *118:* 106–113 (1974).

Sturelid, S. and Kihlman, B.A.: Lysergic acid diethylamide and chromosome breakage. Hereditas *62:* 259–262 (1969).

Swift, M.: Fanconi's anaemia in the genetics of neoplasia. Nature, Lond. *230:* 370–373 (1971).

Swift, M.R. and Hirschhorn, K.: Fanconi's anemia. Inherited susceptibility to chromosome breakage in various tissues. Ann. intern. Med. *65:* 496–499 (1966).

Szabo, K.T.: Teratogenic effect of lithium carbonate in the foetal mouse. Nature, Lond. *225:* 73–75 (1970).

Tjio, J.H. and Levan, A.: The chromosome number of man. Hereditas *42:* 1–6 (1956).

Tjio, J.H.; Pahnke, W.N., and Kurland, A.A.: LSD and chromosomes – a controlled experiment. J. amer. med. Ass. *210:* 849–856 (1969).

Tobin, J.M. and Tobin, J.M.: Mutagenic effects of LSD-25 in *Drosophilia melanogaster.* Dis. nerv. Syst., suppl. *30:* 47–52 (1969).

Trautner, E.M.; Pennycuik, P.R.; Morris, R.J.H.; Gershon, S., and Shankly, K.H.: The effect of prolonged sub-toxic lithium ingestion on pregnancy in rats. Austr. J. exp. Biol. *36:* 305–321 (1958).

Valenti, C.: Discussion of *Jarvik:* Cytogenetic aspects of psychopathology; in *Zubin and Shagass* Neurobiological aspects of psychopathology, pp. 275–280 (Grune & Stratton, New York 1969).

Vesell, E.S.; Page, J.G., and Passananti, T.G.: Genetic and environmental factors affecting ethanol in man. Clin. Pharmacol. Ther. *12:* 192–201 (1971).

Warren, R.J.; Rimoin, D.L., and Sly, W.S.: LSD exposure *in utero.* Pediatrics *45:* 466–469 (1970).

Wright, T.L.; Hoffman, L.H., and Davies, J.: Teratogenic effects of lithium in rats. Teratology *4:* 151–156 (1971).

Zellweger, H.: Anticonvulsants during pregnancy. A danger to the developing fetus? Clin. Pediat. *13:* 338–345 (1974).

Zellweger, H.; McDonald, J.S., and Abbo, G.: Is lysergic acid diethylamide a teratogen? Lancet *ii:* 1066–1068 (1967).

Zelson, C.; Rubio, E., and Wasserman, E.: Neonatal narcotic addiction: 10 year observation. Pediatrics *48:* 178–189 (1971).

Dr. *S.S. Matsuyama,* Veterans Administration Hospital (Brentwood), *Los Angeles, Calif.* (USA)